The Seductive Art of Japanese Bondage

The Seductive Art of Japanese Bondage

by Midori
photographed by Craig Morey

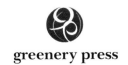

greenery press

Photography: Craig Morey

Illustrations: Jack Cleveland

Cover design: DesignTribe

Cover hair and makeup: Mark Katz

Published in the United States by Greenery Press, 1447 Park Ave., Emeryville, CA 94608, www.greenerypress.com.

ISBN 1-890159-38-7

Contents

Acknowledgments and Thank Yous...

Huge thanks and love go out to Michael and Huck for enduring this whole book birthing process and their ever-strong support. I am ever grateful to Layne Winklebleck of Spectator magazine, Karen at QSM, Kim Airs of Grand Opening and Janet and Patrick of Greenery Press for encouraging me to write and teach. Eternal thanks for the true friendship and research opportunities to Gumby. The inspiration that Michael Manning gave me is as precious as jewels from magical worlds. May my rope work always honor my teachers Lou Duff, Kaye Buckley, Wolf G, Mr. Nagaike, Mr. Randa Mai and Tony DeBlase. My research on historical material and web sources was supported greatly by Tiger from LA, Skye, historical review by Rita, editing help from Bonnie. Thank you so much to all the wonderful models who make this book so sexy: Bonnie, Lisa, Michelle, Tchukon, Nurse Nasty, Sigma, illustration model Bailey, and special thanks to our cover model Dita. Dr. Bill was kind enough to let us use his beautiful home as a photo location. A special deep bow of gratitude to the hospitality, generosity and kindness of Mr. Yanno and Mr. Feldman. I have and will always count on the wonderful inspiration and best conversations with the guys that I think of my favorite uncles of kink, Joseph Bean, Dr. Robert Lawrence and Ira Levine.

And last but certainly not least, all the people I've had the pleasure to bind!

Section One: The Heart

Introduction

Welcome to the pleasures of Japanese-style rope bondage!

For many years, individuals and small groups in the West enjoyed the rather esoteric sensual art of Japanese rope bondage. In recent years, however, there's been a surge of interest in this style of erotic restraint. This is a natural extension of globalization and growth in the new information technology: the ubiquitous Internet, through which any new technology seems to find its way quickly into the realm of sexual expression and erotic exploration.

The Internet, especially post-World Wide Web, has been a boon to the sexually curious. Not only has BDSM made its first few steps out of its leather-lined closet, but today the players are able to look beyond homegrown kink to discover cross-cultural adventures that can enhance their sensuality. Many have delighted in their discovery of severe Germanic rubber play, others have discovered body modification from the South Pacific, and still others have encountered the pleasure of Japanese rope bondage.

Before the wildfire spread of information on the Web, rope bondage techniques in the West, whether in the style of Bob Bishop, John Willie, Tony DeBlase, Japanese or otherwise, had generally been passed from person to person. As Joseph Bean, writer and curator of the Leather Archives and Museum (located in Chicago and serving the world), has pointed out, in the American leather/kink community of the late 20th Century up to the advent of the Internet, the knowledge of specific play techniques was often carefully guarded: mastery of a special skill made a particular top more attractive to approach for play. Some people would apprentice with a knowledgeable player, others would learn in small-scale classes held by the early SM societies such as The Eulenspeigel Society and the Society of Janus. Still others experimented with replicating images from difficult-to-find bondage magazines.

Even today, in the age of the Internet and the proliferation of publicly accessible SM classes, many still choose to learn by these methods. I am one of these people. Perhaps out of stubbornness, a touch of the Luddite, or perhaps due to a preference for the hands-on method of learning, I came to learn rope bondage face-to-face and skin-to-rope. My first attempts at combining rope and sex were also my first explorations of partnered sexual pleasures.

Back in my Berkeley undergraduate days, a lover and I somehow got the idea to take turns tying each other up during sex. In our aged co-op apartment we had set up a cheap futon on a plywood platform resting on cinder blocks. From each corner cinderblock snaked frayed ropes just long enough to wrap around wrists and ankles. It was clumsy, to be sure, but it was fun! In those feverish nights of passion we both learned the pleasure of bondage and the feel of the rope digging into flesh as we devoured each other.

As my interest in this art grew, I had the pleasure of discovering the sexual underground of San Francisco. Here I learned and voraciously absorbed knowledge and experience. I began my journey as a bottom, the one being bound. Of course I found great pleasure in that, but later, as a top, I also came to understand that without the knowledge of being in the rope, I would not have been able to fathom the inner experience of those I bound.

I set out to learn from as many people as I could. I took public and private classes and tutorials from many accomplished rope bondage artists, such as Lou Duff and Wolf G. I learned from those who had learned from Tony DeBlase and other bondage enthusiasts. I apprenticed to Mistress Kaye Buckley, who had spent time as a submissive and bondage performer in Japan in years past. I had the pleasure of learning from Mr. Nagaike, a rope master from Japan, as well as visiting and observing Mr. Randa Mai in Tokyo. Of course, the arena that truly sharpened my skills was the hours, nights and days spent playing with fabulous tops and wonderful bottoms.

My passion for rope comes from other influences as well. Born and raised in Japan, with its unique artistic aesthetics, its deep connections with the art of tying and wrapping, and its profoundly sensual culture, certainly influenced me heavily. (We'll touch lightly on the nature of Japanese aesthetics later.)

Encountering Japanese rope bondage as an adult in the U.S. gave me a sense of being reunited with something ancient in my heritage. The feel of the rope touched something in my soul.

About the same time that I was exploring rudimentary rope bondage in the bedroom, I also spent time in military service, where I came to trust rope for my life. A senior noncommissioned officer showed me how to make a rappelling seat out of rope. With blind trust and youthful foolhardiness I threw myself over the side of walls, secured only by my own rope harness. In Airborne training, I relied on the tensile strength of the cords to keep me floating safely several hundred feet above ground.

Shortly after my military service, I began white-water rafting. There, through the tutelage of more experienced rafters, I learned how to rig the equipment tightly onto the boat and relied on the ropes in the throw bags to get us out of life-threatening situations. Thus, my appreciation, trust and fondness for rope ware set deeply into my heart.

Having shown you my path of studies, now I have to confess my apprehensions in penning this book. For all the years of my passion for rope, I am still learning. Yes, I have taken my own rope *deshi* (apprentices) and have taught classes on this topic across the States. Still, as I took on this book, I was acutely aware that I am not one of the masters that I so admire across the Pacific Ocean. Thus, as one who considers herself still very much on the learning path, I am apprehensive. I would not want to fail to teach well to others what my teachers have taught me so well.

I also feel some sense of apprehension when I realize that Japanese rope bondage, even with my publicly accessible classes, is very much a personal art for me. When I teach others, it is very much a part of my intimate self that I share. In addition, I feel responsible to be there in person, to give them the teaching that only the hands-on approach can give. Yet I've encountered a great thirst for information that is beyond my capacity to teach one-on-one.

I am also concerned about the quality and safety of the various sources of information that are out on the Internet today. Perhaps it would be irresponsible for me to cling to the old methods of teaching out of nostalgia, thus failing to give safe and accurate information to a broader audience that's actively seeking it....

Thus, the time seems to have come to make a book available for the Western readers beyond the pretty glossy photo books. I hope to share with you what I have learned so far so that you may enjoy the pleasures of this particular eroticism. With luck, this will be my first of a series of books as I continue to grow and learn. Although I might not be one of the senior *nawashis* (rope masters) of Japan, I am uniquely suited to be your cultural ambassador of kink.

Let me first share with you a few trade secrets...

The Japanese rope bondage, often referred to as *shibari*, that you see in those beautifully produced glossy coffee table books from Japan, is a bit different from the bondage that we'll be enjoying. Don't worry – I won't be watering down the authenticity for you. Rather, what I will show is Japanese-style rope bondage for real play and accommodating very real Western bodies and practical play concerns.

The conditions for those dramatic photo shoots are considerably different from that of most private play scenes. First of all, their locations might have serious equipment advantage to which you and I might not have access, such as electric winches, hoists and even cranes for the more spectacular outdoor shots. Then there are the petite, feather-light and impossibly flexible young professional bondage models, who come from a culture that values physical endurance as a form of art and discipline. Now add the platoon-sized cast and crew for these shoots, who help to take care of the details that normally the top would have to worry about single-handedly. Thus, the *nawashi* can afford to focus on creating a beautiful, if excruciating, suspension bondage position, keeping the model in that form just long enough for the veteran art photographer to grab some delicious shots. Then, at the signal of the *nawashi*, three or four big guys move in and hoist up the straining model to a comfortable position while the rope master undoes the suspension ties and lowers her gently.

So, don't feel badly if you're not able to replicate what you see in classic Japanese bondage photos or that when you do, you or your partner isn't able to stay in that position for more than a few minutes. Remember that we have our own advantages that these shoots and performances don't: we have the luxury of privacy, intimacy and time.

For this reason, we've chosen to show the poses in this book on a wide range of bodies. Our models range in body type from flexible and slender to muscular and chunky, and in age from early 20s to mid-40s – each stunningly attractive in his or her own way, and each showing ways to adapt the classic poses for different bodies and desires.

We've also chosen, in this book, to stick to basic techniques. With the seven poses shown here, and the several supplemental options and ideas for each one, any reasonably creative person can while away many happy and sexy hours experimenting with different combinations and augmentations. If this book meets with a positive reception, I will probably do a more advanced bondage book later on.

I also must address the issues of pronouns and the fictitious characters in this book. Japanese rope bondage is a pleasure that spans gender and orientation. Any consenting adult can find sweet pleasure in it. Sure, some bondage might be specific to particular genitalia or body forms, but the intelligent reader will easily be able to make the minor alterations necessary to apply it to another body. Therefore you'll find this book peppered with fluid references to the gender of the players. If a particular scene's gender doesn't suit your preference, feel free to change the pronouns to your liking.

The techniques shown in this book are but a few of infinite possibilities. As with any other art, take what you will from these pages, add your own style, experimentation and make it your own. This is simply a starting point.

I hope that this book will provide you with fun, pleasure and many nights of delightful exploration. As with any author, I would be delighted to hear your thoughts and comments!

Your ambassador to kinky pleasures,
Fetish Diva Midori

Beauty and Japanese Rope Bondage

So much of the allure of Japanese rope bondage is the sensual visual beauty of the bound. Simply reducing the submissive's mobility with rope is not enough. Nor is using bondage to enhance sex games. The rope must create visual pleasure for the one binding, the one bound, and any onlookers.

The effect of aesthetic appeal on the scene can be tremendous. As the rope slides onto one bottom's willing flesh, she is inspired by her own beauty as the ravished heroine of her own erotic epic. Another glows in the knowledge that his physique is enhanced and accentuated by the ropes, even as his captive fantasy is realized. Tops may find satisfaction and a surge of sensual power as their creative erotic vision is realized... and find their arousal growing even greater as they behold the sexual beauty of their lovers.

The aesthetics of bondage are what make the difference between a good scene and a great scene. They separate the technically skilled top from the artistic top. Beautiful bondage can make a happy bottom into an elated bottom. How is it so?

I have often found that the bottom with a sexual and physical lust for bondage also has a keen appreciation for the creativity and beauty of the work. Simply binding her efficiently will probably satisfy her physical longing: the bottom is happy, the top is happy and the scene is good.

However, at this point it's primarily the bottom's physical needs that have been met... leaving many other senses yet to be stimulated.

Lovers and SM players are inherently restless seekers of heightened experience. Knowing this, the insightful top weaves into the experience a sense of style and visual beauty beyond common bondage. With this attention, the bottom's mind is also engaged in the appreciation of bondage. She is sensually self-aware that her body is being made into a thing of beauty, pleasing both her and her top. She is more fully engaged in the moment and the experience Even as her spirit flies in the ropes, this aesthetic edge helps her imagination take flight as well. The top has now successfully orchestrated an environment in which all the bottom's senses and awareness have been heightened and are absolutely in the moment: a good scene has become a great scene.

Japanese rope bondage contains an artistic element beyond that of erotic fulfillment and scene pragmatism. Its artistic heart is much like that of *Ikebana* (Japanese flower arrangement), *Bonsai* (miniature tree sculpting) and Japanese architecture. Take the natural ingredient, apply to it the artist's interpretation distilling nature's patterns... thus producing a symbolized homage to the balance and grace of natural forces. Like *Ikebana*, which understands, incorporates and represents the drama of seasons, Japanese rope bondage understands, incorporates and represents the drama of fantasy and sexual desire.

Instead of plunging into a lengthy discussion of the aesthetic theory of Japanese eros relative to Japanese fine art, let's consider a few basic elements of style in *shibari* to get you started.

Elements of Aesthetic Rope

Little things really make a difference in the final beauty of the work. To the uninitiated eye it may not be apparent why, out of two nearly identical bondages with the same pose and construction, one seems more pleasing than the other. It's likely that the more pleasing one has consistent elements of style in the details. Here are some details to be concerned about...

Symmetry. The human body is generally symmetrical along each side of a vertical axis. The eyes, limbs and curves of the body are generally the same on the left as on the right. Our minds tend to find this pleasing and harmonious. When there's a considerable difference along this perceived axis,

we find this unsettling and displeasing. (Imagine Quasimodo or Batman's Two-Face.) The same goes for rope bondage. You'll see this particularly in such body harnesses as the Tortoise Shell *(Kikkou)*, also known as the Diamond *(Hishigata)*, an excellent example of visually pleasing vertical symmetry.

At the smallest level, you want to achieve symmetry in the direction that you tie a knot or loop the rope over another. While this might seem too minute a detail to concern yourself with, it does make a difference in the beauty of the rope. Each time you bind with rope and work on a form that's based on lateral symmetry, pay attention to the directions of the knots on both the left side and the right side. Learning to move with both hands whenever possible will help you to achieve this goal as well.

If on the left side you loop a horizontal rope from the left to right, over a vertical rope and bring it under it, heading back to the left, then on the right side you'll also loop the corresponding horizontal rope from the right to left, over a vertical rope and bring it under it, heading back to the right. Soon you'll find creating symmetrical knots has become second nature.

To a lesser degree, horizontal symmetry is important as well. This happens at a smaller scale in more subtle manifestations. You might see this in the symmetry of the top and bottom halves of a diamond in a harness, or in the number of bands of rope above and under the breast. Sometimes you'll find it in thematic echoes along a horizontal axis, such as a mirror image repetition of a diamond above and below the waistline.

Even tension. The bondage looks best when there's an even tension on the ropes when you've finished tying the whole piece. There is a sense of completeness and finesse to the viewer and the viewed. Even as the body shifts and moves, whether to enjoy the sensuality of the rope for its own sake or under the stimulation of other play, ropes laid evenly tend to move, slack and stretch in unison. No singular part will feel or look as if it's out of control.

Beyond the visual beauty, consistent tension throughout the bondage is safer, and makes the experience feel better for the bound. We'll discuss this issue further in Step By Step: Analysis of a Scene on p. 21.

There are ties where you'll have to begin with a considerable amount of slack to the rope. Do this when you anticipate that you'll add other ropes later on to tighten up existing lines. A good example of this is the Tortoise Shell Body Harness *(Kikkou)*. The first set of ropes along the length of the body go on loosely. As the tying continues, the horizontal lines tighten up the slack. If the first set of ropes were laid down in their final tension, then the additional horizontal lines would only make them much tighter, possibly tighter than is safe.

Conversely, if you find that you've allowed too much slack in a line, you can use other lines to take up the slack with counter-directional tension, thus providing better tension.

Twists. Unintentional twists in the rope make the bondage look sloppy. Where the ropes are wrapped or coiled around several times to form a band, don't let the lines twist over each other haphazardly. Conscientiously lay the rope and then run your hand over the finished band to feel for the smooth evenness. Adjust where necessary.

As with the discussion above on even tension, avoiding haphazard twists is not only pretty, it's better for the bound body. Smooth bands serve to support the body, whereas the twisted lines create uneven areas of pressure. At best, these areas are uncomfortable and may lead to bruises or abrasions. Some also feel that this unevenness might negatively affect pressure points along the meridians described in various Asian healing traditions.

As with any rule, there are exceptions, and twists in the line is one of these. Later you'll see when an intentional twist might prove quite advantageous and pleasurable.

Balance, Eye Flow and Intentional Asymmetry. A sense of movement and drama can be expressed even in stillness. Paintings, flower arrangements and other art that inspire often bring our attention to one point, then seemingly effortlessly lead our gaze through a flow. Hokusai's famous woodblock print "The Great Wave Off Kanagawa," of the enormous wave framing the serene Mount Fuji, moves our gaze in a dynamic circle, leaving us with a sense of exhilaration and awe. Incorporating the geometry of balance and degrees of symmetry in the overall form of the bondage can enhance a sense of stability or motion.

Consider the image of a triangle. When it rests on its side it appears grounded and stable. Images of Mount Fuji, a favorite subject of Edo era artists, incorporate this triangular form to portray permanence, gravity and immobility. Now consider the general form of the *Agura* position (p. 111), where the sub sits with his legs crossed on the floor. The general outline is of this stable triangle. Its center of gravity is lower and it is laterally symmetrical. This gives an impression of great stability and immobility while being visually balanced. Our gaze moves down from the head and shoulder directly to the base formed by the legs, and stays there.

When the triangle is inverted, resting on one of its points, it looks precariously balanced. If that triangle is then tilted a bit, there's a sense that it's in mid-motion, about to tilt at any moment. The partial suspension shown on page 129 is an excellent representation of this aesthetic. The head, the raised leg and the grounded leg form the inverse triangle outline. The gaze moves from the head, along the torso to the raised leg, down the grounded leg and then back up again to the upper frame of the photo. The center of the gravity of this image is higher up and the gaze is always kept

moving, adding to the sense of precariousness of this position. If you raised the suspended leg much higher, then allow the head and upper body to dip down further, you would now have the tilted triangle. The sweep of the raised leg to the torso also creates an elegant arc reminiscent of Hokusai's Wave. In this position the gaze moves from one end of the arc and beyond, as if the eyes were following an invisible curve flowing beyond the head and leg.

The use of the triangular form is just one shape to help consider balance and flow of the bondage form. There are other examples of geometry of balance and degrees of symmetry. The *Gyakuebi*, or the Hog-Tie (p. 141), is an oval or ellipse on its side, the body harnesses work on and around a rectangle, etc. While the regular Open Leg Crab (*Kaikyaku Kani*) (p. 47) is fundamentally a stable triangle, if you throw one leg out the opposite direction, then you have a slanted L where the gaze flows from the head, to one knee, to the other foot that's pointing out, and then beyond. The eye flows as if you were gazing on the movement of a waterfall or the flowing position of the seated Kannon, the deity of mercy.

This last reference to the seated Kannon actually betrays one of my secret sources of inspiration for bondage forms – the art museums. I enjoy studying the statues and paintings, particularly of Asian images of deities as well as the Symbolists of 19th century Europe, to find inspiration in the beauty of the human body so I can bring that grace into my bondage. I will often position my submissives without rope into the same position as sculptures, perhaps that of an Indian temple dancer sculpture I saw at the Sackler Gallery, or the White Tara at the San Francisco Asian Art Museum. Then I will use my powers of visualization to figure out how I will use my knowledge of rope bondage to honor and reflect that beauty now manifested in my play partner.

Gusto. The rope that goes on with gusto will look decisively placed, strong and dominant. The rope laid tentatively will appear indecisive, weak and half-hearted, and thus less inspiring. This "gusto" and confidence only comes with time and practice. Initially it's best to concentrate on the fundamental techniques, safety and beauty. When this starts to feel like second nature, you're ready to apply the ropes with decisiveness and speed. This is when you start to feel the rope move by its own wishes from your hands. If you've ever looked at the dramatic bondage photos in the tradition of Ito, you'll see these bold moves. Oddly enough, at this level of skill you'll notice that the ropes may not always be on in perfect smoothness and the bondage might even appear rough and unruly. This is the accomplished artist's hand at work, which is focused on the drama and intent on creating an image that conveys a sense of struggle and a story.

Japanese rope bondage is both a living art form and a vital expression of sexuality. It's an ever changing, expressive and dynamic collaboration between the top, bottom and the rope. It's not frozen in tradition. Learn the basics thoroughly. Learn the rules well so you know how to break them beautifully with mindful purpose.

A Brief Folkloric History of the Rope in Japan

As with most aspects of SM, the history of Japanese rope bondage is murky. Reliable information is often difficult to locate, and the most interesting data is frequently anecdotal or folkloric. Having said this, I will share with you some highlights of the information I've amassed through conversations and research, as well as lessons and impressions from my Japanese heritage.

The relationship of the Japanese, rope and tying objects is a long one, possibly as old as the Japanese civilization itself. It can be found as far back as the Jomon period (10,000 BCE to 300 BCE), where rope played a significant role in cultural expression. The term Jomon literally means "rope pattern," after their distinctive rope-patterned pottery (Figure 1). From antiquity to today, Japanese religious ceremonies involve heavy use of rope and ties to symbolize connections among people and the divine, as well as to delineate sacred space and time.

The quintessential nature of rope and the art of tying resonate from the sacred arena to the secular. Up until recent Westernization it seemed that just about everything in Japan was somehow tied together. Take the basic garment, the kimono.

It does not have a single button or hook, but rather is closed by ritually tying standardized fabric shapes to the body. The act of tying customized the clothing to the wearer. Even military battle-armor consisted of panels of lacquered wood elegantly tied together (Figure 2). Gifts – to the gods, to one's social superior or to a friend – no matter how humble the content, had to be intricately wrapped and elaborately tied.

These conventions hold true even today. Consider, for example, the tradition of prettily and functionally wrapping goods

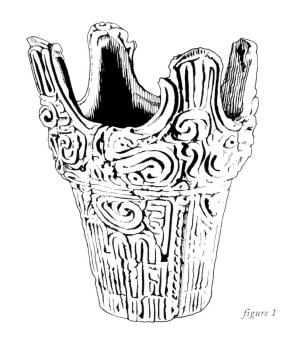

figure 1

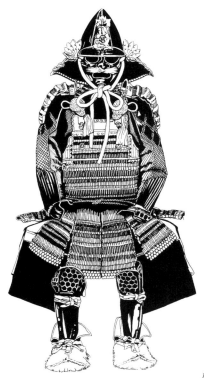

figure 2

in a square cloth *(furoshiki)*, the intricate cord tying on packages *(mizuhiki)* or even the special ways in which gift money is wrapped. These are all examples of the Japanese culture's need to properly wrap items with the occasion and appropriate respect in mind. Such objects are not to be handled thoughtlessly and must be presented in a manner pleasing to the beholder.

Elaborate tying of objects can be found in unexpected places in modern Japan. I remember being at a SM video shoot in Tokyo where I noticed that the camera operator had stabilized the monitor as well as the lights using rope bondage just as impressive as the bondage on the model's soft flesh. It was something so natural to him that he didn't even think twice about it.

Considering how the art of tying and binding is deeply embedded into Japanese culture, it should not be surprising that it

also became an integral part of battle techniques – both a martial art and a tool of incarceration. During the Japanese "Dark Ages" of the Sengoku/Muromachi period (approx. 1467 - 1600), a long period of peace and prosperity was shattered, leaving the nation torn by brutal warfare. In this climate, among a multitude of other warrior arts, the martial arts of capturing, transporting, interrogating and torturing prisoners developed. *Tasuki-dori* and *Hobaku-jutsu* are traditional techniques for capturing and detaining an opponent while *Hojo-jutsu* is a technique for using rope on an opponent once detained. It's widely believed that our current Japanese erotic rope restraint techniques originated during this period.

At this point, the Western reader may be wondering why other materials for incarceration and detentions common to the Indo-European cultures, such as leather, metal and wood, were not used. Economics and resource availability played a great part in this difference. In an island nation bordered by a thin ribbon of cultivatable land, it was more important to allocate that land to rice paddies than the more resource- and land-intensive cattle-raising. Thus leather, the byproduct of cattle culture, was a scarce commodity for common folk.

Similar problems with technology, availability and resource limited the use of metal: although the Japanese perfected sword-making, the use of metal in the mass scale that would have allowed for the common use of metal fetters was not feasible in Japan's middle ages.

While wood is used in images of incarceration, bamboo appears more frequently. Abundant, quick-growing, easy to harvest and diverse in its usage, bamboo became a practical and common material for bondage as well as many other uses. Similarly, materials for rope-making were cheap and abundant. Under these conditions, rope was the natural tool for incarceration in times of war.

It was during the Edo period (1600-1868) that the Tokugawa government instituted unique political policies of peacekeeping, thereby making the warring days a thing of the past. The resulting unprecedented nationwide prosperity expanded the mercantile class and lifted it to hitherto unseen levels of wealth and power. It was at this point that the family tree of rope arts made a huge split.

One branch maintained its purpose as a disciplined yet pragmatic method of criminal/prisoner management. The standard martial art forms were polished and perfected by different schools, becoming highly codified with many subtle variations of rope colors and methods of tying to reflect the rank of the captured, level of crime, season of the year, etc. Edo seems to have been the time when the martial art of rope approached the finesse of the decorative arts. There are still schools of martial arts today, as well as some police uses of rope, that are direct descendants of these practices.

While the first branch of the rope bondage family tree reinforced and extended traditional martial art forms, the second branch grew in a completely different direction. The prosperity of the Edo period resulted in a growing and affluent middle class with an increasing demand for entertainment and gratification. Images of rope bondage in different media helped to meet these needs.

One of the most popular entertainments was the Kabuki theater. While today the Kabuki theater is considered a classical Japanese art form, back then it was not far removed from its roots as a troupe of traveling performers. Kabuki's evolution from mass entertainment with a rowdy pit to high art parallels that of Shakespeare's plays at the original Globe Theatre. Like Shakespeare, it was very much the commoner's theater, full of bawdy images including *nureba* (romance and sex scenes) and *semega* (torture scenes).

The popularity of Kabuki was further enhanced by significant improvements in wood block printing technology. There was soon a thriving industry of printed kabuki tie-in products for the fans. Leaflets and images were printed and sold, depicting the popular actors and plays, often seen in particularly hot scenes from the playbill.

From these humble, commercial beginnings came the now well-respected art form of the *Ukiyoe*, or images of the floating world. Sexual images *(nureba)* and torment scenes *(semega)* were popular fare and ultimately gave birth to a new breed of mass media erotic artists. This process was hardly unique to Japan. Consider Victorian England and Europe in the same period, another place where the consuming middle class thrived. They too enjoyed a boon of mass distribution of sexual images in early photographs, illustrations and stories. The U.S. equivalent of this phenomenon was the mid-20th century flourishing of pin-up magazines and true crime pulp novels with bound women on the covers.

Many of the famous *Ukiyoe* artists took apprentices to extend their popularity and commercial viability by continuing their stylistic legacy. One of the last practitioners of this *Ukiyoe*-style, consumer-oriented popular art was Seiu Ito (1882–1961). Although born in the Meiji Restoration era, his style was firmly rooted in the Edo woodblock print tradition. Not only was he a traditional artist, a recognized *semega* master, he also had a personal interest in SM spurred by tales of captive princesses told to him by his mother when he was nine or ten years old. His artistic eye for sensual aesthetics and this personal sexual interest led him to take his first photographs of "punished women" in 1919. I see this as the dawn of the modern form of erotic Japanese rope bondage.

By the mid 1920s there were already a few sadomasochistic erotic photo magazines in circulation featuring Ito's photos. It seems that he was the primary creative force behind these publications. Much like today's artists who are inspired by the computer and the Internet, back then the new technology of photography spurred the artistic and erotically inclined to new levels of expression. Ito's stylistic influence still deeply colors contemporary commercial severe rope bondage *(kinbaku)* imagery. The bound women's mussed or disheveled hair was his trademark. In these striking, almost ghostly images, the women had expressions of wistful suffering and aroused shame. Look at today's highly produced and popularized images and you'll still feel his spectral hand guiding their vision.

After World War II, war-torn Japan slowly built up its economy and once again a middle class emerged hungry for entertainment and stimulation. In the early 1950s a number of erotic bondage photo magazines appeared, the most prominent of which was "Kitan Club" ("Strange Tales Club") in 1952. The 1950s also saw the birth of the bondage photo clubs, not unlike those of Irving Klaw and Bettie Page in the US. The new mass-market SM/bondage magazine genre enjoyed a modest boom, infusing the new medium with sexuality, power exchange fantasies and aesthetics familiar to the Japanese from the previous century. At this time bondage performance clubs started to pop up as well, featuring rope masters combining stunning rope bondage work now called *shibari*, dramatic suspension and high theatrical energy. During the 1960s a period of social moralism swept the country, driving the images, magazines and bondage fans underground for a while, only to re-emerge with even greater verve in the late 1970s under a more permissive social climate.

Today, while Japanese rope bondage and SM are still considered to be somewhat "underground," both are thriving at an unprecedented level. Many sexual magazines portray bondage, humiliation, etc., with many images echoing the rope-based martial arts of the medieval era combined with an *Ukiyoe* sensual aesthetic.

It is also worth observing that while the ranks of Japanese dominants have traditionally been male, the changing role of women in modern Japan has created a huge influx of female dominants or Queens *(Joh-sama)* into the published media, theater and rope bondage dominance. Like the West, there's been an increasing crossing over of kinky, SM and fetish images into the mainstream media and social consciousness, giving a new spark of renegade glamor to the rope masters and mistresses of Japan today.

The Seduction

Him:

I let the rope run through my hands as I gaze upon her curving form. Methodically I fold the rope in two, resting the center point in my right hand, as I breathe to find focus. I watch her as she slowly and purposefully stretches her graceful limbs. She is beautiful. She gives me the gift of her body. As I admire her, the vision of her bound body forms in my mind. The patterns emerge. For this moment there's only the two of us in this world. Tonight I will hold her at the edge of ecstasy…

Her skin is cool to my touch but her face is flushed with desire. I grasp her shoulders firmly and she surrenders with grace to my guidance. Slowly I find her wrists, feeling the tension slip from her fingertips. Her eyes close and I can see her slipping into sensual submission. Her serene smile and light touches on my skin let me know that it's all good. I feel her love flow through me, giving me new power. A quick controlled move and I've pulled her arms into a more disciplined posture. A sigh-gasp escapes her lips. Erotic…

Her:

I stand naked before him, aroused… ready for our adventure. I shed my clothes and worries of the day. I can smell the sweet cut-grass smell of the hemp rope. The scent alone can take me there. I let my soul be naked to the moment. I watch him caress the rope through his hands… soon it'll be me in his hands.

With firm guiding hands he moves my body. I yield to his desire so that my desires may be freed. Swiftly he takes my arms and binds them behind me. A well-practiced motion, now so ingrained in him that it's effortless and seemingly without premeditation. Even in his apparent casualness, I feel his total focus of his being upon me. Right now there's only the two of us. He holds me from behind and my wrists turn freely to caress his taut, naked belly.

With a quick tug of the rope my arms are jacked up and his soft loving touch suddenly turns decisive and cool. Something deep inside me starts to melt. The new tension in my muscles heightens my awareness of my own body…

Him:

...dominance surges through me. I swiftly wrap the ropes around her arms, under her breasts and then above. Taking the time with the underarm hitch, I slide a finger between the rope and the delicate skin as not to pinch her while cinching the line. Moving my hands in tandem, I slide the lines over her shoulder, placing two pairs of perfectly symmetrical half-hitches at her cleavage. Letting the rope fall from my hands, I stop to admire her, softly caressing the tender undercurve of her supple breasts. This is just the moment of calculated calm needed for next bit of drama. I love leading this dance, quick, quick, slow, slow... soft, sensual, hard and back again. One hand still sweetly playing with her breast, the other hand reaches to the loose rope. One quick yank up, and then down, the breast ropes tighten down. I'm rewarded with another sweet sigh-gasp.

Now that I have her wide-eyed focus again, I lead her down fully onto her feet with the ropes, firmly grounding her senses back into her body. A broad grin of satisfaction crosses my face. Resuming a more measured pace, I tie off the lines above the wrists and reach for more rope. Tying it into the chest knot, I measure out three overhand knots onto the doubled line... one below her ribs, one above her mound and one carefully resting on her clit hood just behind the pelvic bone. Pleased with my perfect placement, I slide...

Her:

... a bit like the muscle tension right before I come.

The ropes seem to fly out of his fingers, dancing to his will and snaking around me. The ropes kiss and lick me all over, sometimes hot scalding bites and sometimes sweet gentle strokes. Soon my arms are bound down tightly. I love the way he turns me to wrap me, the way he takes charge of my body. He gazes into me and I'm awash in his tenderness. Unexpected light strokes to my breasts, now awakened by the ropes, send a shudder up my spine, making my vulva pulse.

My body purrs into his touch, melting. Without warning, a fiery flash explodes in my chest and fades out to the tightness of a strong embrace, and I realize that he's cinched my breast in even tighter. I'm pulled up onto the balls of my feet, back arching back as he leans into me. I breathe in his power. Pressing his strong body into mine, he slowly lowers me back down onto my feet. His breath hot on my temple as I nuzzle into his neck, feeling the sureness of the moment as I steady myself back onto my feet. The ropes begin to fly from his fingers again, and I close my eyes to enjoy each touch. Oh, he's a devil! I can feel the clit-knot and I know what that means! There'll be more pleasure to come; that's for sure! I practically shriek in delight as he slides the rope along my pussy. In brisk measured...

Him:

... the ropes along her swelling vulva, then work the rope from her back side to front and back again, creating a series of firm diamond shapes on her body, befitting my treasured beauty. With each length of the rope I am wrapping myself around her. The rope is the extension of my desire, lust and love for her. I see the lines sink into her curves. I know what the ropes are tasting, that sweet honey fig taste. For a moment, as I gaze upon her, it's me that sinking into her flesh.

Grasping the cluster of rope in the middle of her back like a handle, I give a gentle shove and throw her off balance a bit. With the other hand pressed into her chest I guide her down onto her knees. She yields with grace like water flowing over rocks. With my hand still on the back ropes, I shift her to get better at her legs. As I spread her thighs I see that the ropes in her sex are darkened with moisture. Good. One rope on each leg, I bind the lower leg to the thigh, leaving a bit of line free. With each leg's mobility effortlessly restricted, I take the loose lines and attach the free ends to the arm ropes. Tugging the lines through to a clean simple knot, I pry her legs apart – a ripe peach split open ready for the devouring. I swallow the hungry impulse to consume right there and then. No, I have a purpose tonight... I can wait.

Out of her sight, I fish out the vibrator from the nightstand. Not the ever-favorite...

Her:

... moves my torso is quickly embraced in a web of rope. He lets me stand free for a moment, letting me sink into the feeling of the ropes. He watches me as I shift my weight from this side to that, then writhe in the ropes, feeling secure in them, feeling them gently dig into my skin. I feel the slow pressure on my pulsing clit. It makes me squirm even more. With every move I'm aware of him, all around me, as I sway in his rope embrace.

Soon his gaze shifts off me, and he grabs me by the ropes. How easily he moves me! In one move he pushes me off center, then back, assuring me of his control and my safety. I surrender further under his protective power. Am I the sex puppet to his puppet-master tonight? Easily he moves me down onto the soft carpet. He moves my legs this way and that and the ropes fly again. Soon I'm tightly bound and spread open, the ropes digging deeper into my wet lips.

My desire is so transparent to him... Self-consciousness rises under his gaze and my face burns in the flush of embarrassment of how exposed my eagerness for him is. Here and now he will not let me hide my lust. Aroused even more by my own embarrassment, I can do nothing but present my body to his probing gaze. I wallow in my sweet helplessness... although I'm not sure if I'm helpless now in his ropes or in facing my own desires....

Him:

... wall-powered wand, but the simple, slim plastic model. Popping in a couple of fresh batteries, I check the controls. The buzzing sound elicits a low purring moan of expectation from my sweet captive. Cruel chuckles escape my lips as I return to find her flushed and squirming. Approaching her with the vibe I make a move as if to place the pleasure toy on her clit, but instead I move it up her body. Was that a groan of disappointment or anticipation? I slide the vibe just above the knot at her rib and turn the switch on to full power. She cries out her pleasure and quivers and grinds against the ropes. I watch over her ecstatic agony with great satisfaction. It's such a thrill to have the power to create great pleasure and moments of abandon, to control her pleasure so acutely... I'll savor my sweet captive's quivering for a while... and then....

Her:

...I'm spared his burning gaze as he moves across the room. I try to regain even breathing for a moment, but my efforts are in vain. As soon as I exhale for calm I hear the siren-song buzzing of my old vibrator! He teases me and denies my hungry sex of its sweet sensations. Instead he places it on my torso, leaving me puzzled. When he turns it on I find out what a devilishly sweet top he is! Soon the all the ropes are vibrating, every part of me is pulsing and all my entire body is a huge erogenous zone. Waves of pleasure wash over me, building, building, building... to a crest, then receding, only to build again. I strain against the bonds freely, thrashing in my pleasure all that I may. I let the pleasure build up and up and up, losing sense of everything except blind hedonistic pleasure....

I hope you enjoyed this little story and that it whetted your appetite for play! This wasn't simply a titillating way to fill the pages: it's also a sly little instructional. You'll find embedded in the stories above all the essential elements for a hot Japanese rope bondage scene. Now for the play-by-play analysis and how-to, turn to "Analysis of a Scene" on the next page.

Step by Step: Analysis of a Scene

Now you know the historical background, and have read what a play experience can be like. But how do you actually create a steamy scene without feeling like you're doing a Boy Scouts' knot-tying drill?

In this section we'll take a look at some of the elements of scene dynamics embedded in the "Seduction of Rope" chapter on page 17 that made the experience so hot. There is much more involved in creating a fantastic scene than the ability to create beautiful rope patterns on a body.

This section is not intended to dictate how you must conduct a given scene. Rather, this is a method by which I can best share with you some of the details that go into a scene dynamic. Take the information given here and incorporate it as it best suits your needs.

As with any sensual or SM interaction, both the top and the bottom's parts are equally, if differently, important in order to create a fulfilling experience. Let's start with the top's share of the experience:

For the Top:

1. *"I let the rope run through my hands"*
   This is a simple physical action full of meanings and functions. To list a few...

- A skein of rope may have been stored for a short or long period of time. Inconsistent bends or "habits" may be developed in the rope, depending on how long and how it may have been stored. "Bad habits" in the rope will make it move and sit inconsistently on the body. While we like our playmates to be kinky, we don't like it in our rope. Running the rope through the hands allows these kinks to get worked out. I like to do this, not just to open the scene, but with each rope that I uncoil for use.

- It's quite common, even for the most careful players, for the rope to pick up debris during previous play use. Some of these foreign objects, such as splinters, can be quite unpleasant to the bottom, potentially ruining the scene. I know of a person whose rope somehow caught a stray staple somewhere along the way. He had applied the rope to the bottom without knowing this. When time came to remove the rope, the tugging raked the sharp metal end across the bottom's skin, gouging her. If you run the rope lightly through your hands first, you will be able to detect any potential hazard in advance.

- Some ropes age well while others wear out quickly. Eventually, through loving use, all rope will start to fray, unwind or otherwise lose its structural integrity. Running the hands over it will allow you to feel for such inconsistencies. Once you find it, you can decide what to do with it: discard the rope, cut the damaged part and make two or more smaller but usable pieces, or relegate that piece to a less strenuous role in the overall bondage.

- Each rope has a different "burn speed." This is the pace at which the rope running across the skin causes friction unbearable and/or damaging to the skin. Nylon and many other synthetic ropes seem to have a relatively slow burn speed. This means that it only takes a slow pace of the rope running across the skin to feel like a hole being burned through the flesh. Cotton and hemp ropes seem to have a rather high burn speed. If you're using new or unfamiliar rope, you may wish to find out where the burn speed for that line is so you know how to manage it around the bottom to create the exact desired effect. Running the rope through your hands will allow you to find out exactly what the rate and the consequential sensation will be.

- Running the rope through the hands at the beginning of a scene may serve to focus many dominants to the moment, enabling them to be fully present in the experience. Becoming present in the scene experience is not just necessary for the bottom. Tops must do what they need to do to find the state of mind for a fully enjoyable scene, or "head space."

- While effectively setting the tone and head space for the dominant, the visual effect of the top methodically stroking the ropes may be quite profound on the bottom and help him to create his submissive "head space." Many different moods and attitudes might be presented by the top and seen by the bottom: powerful and slightly intimidating, soothing and reassuring, playful, humiliating, sensual or any number of desired attitudes to set the tone for the bottom. A simple act like running the rope through your hands holds the potential for a theatrical visual effect that inspires just the right mood for both players and any other observers.

- While the dominant is doing all the above, the simple act of running the rope through her hands might be buying her the time needed to find inspiration for the moment and the vision of the bondage.

2. *"I can smell the sweet cut grass smell of the hemp rope. The scent alone can take me there."*

These words were from the submissive's narrative, but it's indicative of her past scenes with this top or with others. She has come to associate the unique scent of the hemp rope with the sensual, sexual and magical experience of wonderful rope bondage scenes. While this association could happen by luck and accident, it's more likely that it's happened because of the conscious planning of the insightful top. Creating positive association between key sensory input and pleasures helps to bring the bottom, and often the top as well, into a fully present mindset to enjoy the scene and anticipate pleasure. If you wish, you can think of this as a way to consensually instill a sensual Pavlovian response. This can be done with any of the senses, whether the sound of a key word, the sight of something special, or a particular touch. But scent holds a special place, as scent is an extremely primal memory trigger for us. The hemp rope has a most unique and pleasant scent reminiscent of cut grass, tatami mats or dried hay, making it easy to create this positive sensual association to begin a scene with. This is one of the many reasons I love using hemp rope in Japanese bondage.

3. *"fold the rope in two… the center point in my right hand"*

It is most common in Japanese rope bondage to start with the rope folded in two and beginning the tie at the center point. This allows for time saved in wrapping as well as symmetry in design.

4. *"find focus"*

It is the top's responsibility to be fully present to the experience of the scene with the bottom. We spend so much of our lives living in the past and worrying about the future that we need to treasure the special quality of SM scenes to bring us into the moment. While it's easy to say this and recognize it for its importance, it's not always easy to do. Each top will find his or her way to ground and focus before a scene. You will find your own as well. One of my favorite methods – and I have found other rope dominants report the same – is to take the time to caress the rope as I unfurl the skein. It makes me aware of my skin. More importantly, I have done so at the beginning of so many scenes that by now it's taken on a ritualistic quality. This act for me is now full of purpose and meaning, indicating the time of transition from the mundane to the extraordinary.

Beyond treasuring the rare opportunity to be in the moment, why is it so important for the dominant in the scene to find focus? First, don't underestimate the bottom's ability to sense your presence or lack of presence in the moment. When they find you distracted, it's likely that they won't surrender as deeply as they could have… or worse, will lose respect for you. It's also worth noting that the lack of grounded focus or the distracted mindset of the dominant can lead to critical carelessness or moments of inattentiveness that may cause accidents or injuries.

5. *"she… stretches"*

Bondage can be very physically demanding. To the casual observer it might seem that bondage leaves the bottom unmoving and thus is strictly a physically passive activity. This is hardly the case. While some bondage positions, such as the ornamental body harness, strain the body very little, many Japanese rope bondage positions that derive from methods of interrogation are extremely stressful to the muscles. The body is often placed in unaccustomed positions leading to muscle fatigue, cramps and even exertion of energy to maintain balance.

Many bottoms also delight in the freedom to struggle and feel the full strength of their own body in the ropes. This explosive energy might lead to strains and sprains in the muscle. These sort of unplanned and unpleasant pains can distract or halt an otherwise exciting scene.

It's really easy to reduce the possibility of such interruptions. Approaching the SM play scene as you would any other physically demanding sport might be helpful. A little stretching before the scene on part of the bottom will go a long way to injury prevention. Plenty of hydration helps as well. The top may choose to ask or order the bottom to stretch, depending on the emotional dynamics of the two in the scene.

6. *"vision of her bound body forms in my mind... patterns emerge"*

Take the time to consider how you want the bondage to look. A bit of visualization will allow you to plan the bondage scene effectively. With this vision of how you wish to bind and how the scene will proceed, you'll be able to gather the necessary materials and figure out what kind of tying you'll need to do to achieve your goals. Visualization will also allow you to identify any points of potential physical hazard and plan for them in advance. A

failure to think this through may also cause you to have to redo the bondage mid-scene.

For example, what if you had hoped to have sex at the end the bondage scene and yet you proceed to tie up your partner in a manner that allowed no access to any sexual fun for either of you? You'd have to undo the bondage considerably, losing some steam.

Or suppose you've tied a new bottom into the traditional form with the wrists tied together behind the back and the ropes securing the upper arms to the chest. You begin by tying the wrists together where they cannot be easily undone. You proceed with the scene to create an intricate array of cords that are a pleasure to behold. Two-thirds into completion, however, the bottom's arms start to tingle and you remember that this position can be difficult for many. All you need to do to relieve the bottom's discomfort is to untie the wrists. Unfortunately, you didn't use a quick-release safety tie for the wrists. Now you have to decide between untying the whole bondage or cutting the rope to prevent the bottom from possible injury.

Plan ahead for a scene by taking the time to visualize the position. It'll save you a lot of time in the long run.

7. *"Tonight I will hold her at the edge of ecstasy"*

Know the intent of your scene. Each scene has its own intent, whether clearly stated during negotiation or not. Play partners with a long history may not explicitly discuss goals of a scene before play, but rather read the more subtle cues that they've come to know in each other.

Some scenes with rope bondage are about creating a loving cocoon around the bottom where he can feel warm and safe. Another scene might be about physical endurance and masochism, while another scene might use the bondage to achieve a larger fantasy such as interrogation or captivity games. Sometimes the bondage is used as a prelude for sex, while sometimes the bondage is an end in itself. Deciding on your intent is part of the preparation for the scene, along with visualization mentioned above. Like the visualization, it allows for better planning of the experience, preparation and risk reduction.

8. *"Her skin is cool to my touch"*

At the beginning of the scene I like to lightly touch the bottom's skin, sometimes on the face, sometimes elsewhere, but always making sure to touch the arms and hands. At one level this simple act serves to connect my play partner and me emotionally through the warm physical touch. It's a loving gesture with which to begin the scene. At another level, I am also gauging and noting the baseline skin temperature of my submissive. Some people have naturally warmer or colder skin temperature. Knowing this in advance will help me judge mid-scene if a cold limb might necessitate a change in position or pace of the scene.

9. *"grasp her shoulders firmly"*

When moving a person in bondage, always do so decisively, with a touch that signals clearly what you wish them to do so that they may better yield to your guidance. It's easier for the bottom to determine the direction of guidance applied to the shoulder than to the wrist. Not only does it make it a smoother motion, it enforces their confidence in your dominance and

control of the scene. Also, it's wise to move people by guiding them by their shoulders, upper arms, hips and torso, but generally not by their wrists. Using the wrist to guide a person whose mobility is compromised by the bondage can lead to potential injury.

You will establish psychological dominance by choosing to move the submissive while you bind them instead of moving yourself. It's a subtle but effective touch. It's best to reserve this physical method for psychological dominance when they are steady enough to move safely by themselves.

10. *"Her serene smile and light touches... lets me know that it's all good."*

Always read all the signals that the bottom's giving, whether with words, touch, facial expressions or sound. If you are playing with a person new to you, then make sure to let them know what kind of feedback you need to let you know if the experience at the moment is good or bad for them. You should also find out what feedback they commonly give or are able to give.

11. *"quick controlled move... pulled her arms into a more disciplined posture"*

Firm decisive moves, sometimes punctuated by a quick change in pace such as the one described here, serve to emphasize the emotional dominance and control that the top has over the scene by a clear physical action. Many subs delight in this as much as their dominants do. It's quite dramatic and psychologically effective. It may also serve to bring the bottom back fully into the present if the top suspects their attention might be wavering off the scene. This is different than the wonderful state where the bottom is experiencing a near meditative state induced by the pleasure and rhythm of the ropes, sometimes referred to as being "in the zone."

Be careful, however, not to make the move so exaggerated that it might cause injury. This is especially true with the arms behind the back. A little firmness in the motion is all you need to get the message across.

12. *"wrap the ropes around her arms, under her breasts and then above"*

The bondage discussed in this narrative is a combination of a few of the positions discussed in the other parts of this book. He starts out with the Arm and Chest *(Ushirote munenawa)*, Position 2, then combines this with the ornamental Tortoise Shell Body Harness *(Kikkou)*, Position 3, then finishes it off with the Open Leg Crab *(Kaikyaku kani)*, Position 1.

The bondage positions discussed here are meant to give you a strong foundation in Japanese style rope bondage. I encourage you to master these and then actively combine them to suit your vision and intent.

13. *"slide a finger between the rope and the skin as not to pinch while cinching"*

Sometimes you can just pull the rope freely, at other times you need to be more careful. In this move from the Arm and Chest *(Ushirote munenawa)* position, it's really easy to abrade and pinch the tender skin between the arm and torso, as the space is so tight. In order to prevent this, move the lines slowly. You may also need to slide a finger between the skin and the

moving rope to prevent rope burn. This technique comes in handy on other parts of the skin or when using rope with slow burn speed. Save your bottom's skin from unintentional discomfort so that you may dish out the sensually cruel sensations when you intend to.

14. *"Moving my hands in tandem"*

Since many of the techniques discussed in Japanese bondage use the doubled-over rope technique, often you'll need to split the lines and bind them in symmetrical patterns. Moving both hands in tandem proves to be advantageous for many reasons. It's more efficient and time saving. With some practice you'll find that using both hands will allow you to create bondage with consistent tension and positioning that's difficult to duplicate when tied unilaterally. This bilateral, two-handed bondage action, accompanied with a smooth practiced motion, is often soothingly rhythmic and hypnotic for both the players, enhancing the "head space." Thus, this is one of those little details of bondage skills that make for a better bondage experience overall.

15. *"perfectly symmetrical half hitches"*

As discussed in the Aesthetics chapter, the visual pleasure of Japanese rope bondage is considerably enhanced by paying attention to the symmetry in the placement of the ropes and knots. If a half hitch on one side of the body moves from outside to inside, moving under a perpendicular line, then the corresponding knot should also do the same. Imagine a mirror placed along the axis of the body, or the axis of the bondage, and design it from there. It may be a subtle difference, but when the entire piece is completed, these little touches imperceptibly accumulate to create a visually pleasing experience.

Beyond the satisfaction of visual completeness and balance, the symmetry in knot placement affects the physical perception of sensation and sensual rightness for the bottom. Knots that are obviously asymmetrical will create a sense of something being amiss in the flesh of the bottom. If you appreciate or study pressure points and meridians of the traditional Asian healing arts, you may also be concerned that a pressure point may be affected differently on each side of the body. We will leave the discussion of pressure points and rope bondage for another occasion.

16. *"moment of calculated calm... leading this dance... soft, sensual, hard and back again"*

Understanding the SM scene as a dance shared between two passionate people – a dance with its own rhythm and drama – is not just an element for a good rope bondage scene, it's an essential perspective on any thrilling SM experience. Like a tango, one leads, sets the tone and guides the other through the practiced movements, avoiding obstacles and adding unique flourishes. The follower yields with grace, yet moves equally eloquently with the practiced grace of her own, making the dance possible. While the dancers may be the same, each dance is a new experience.

Keeping this perspective in mind, keep it fresh and keep the rhythm changing. Don't fall into the common trap of monotony in pace or planning. Some of this rhythm will include calculated moments of calm punctuated by physical or emotional

excitement and unpredictability.

17. *"lead her down fully onto her feet"*

If the top intentionally moves the bottom physically or emotionally off balance, it is also her responsibility to bring him fully back to a state of balance. This deepens the trust and confidence of the bottom for the top. It lets him know that she cared for him and is also competent enough to know exactly what's going on for him.

18. *"tie off the lines above the wrists..."* *"Grasping the cluster of rope in the middle of her back..."*

When the rope runs out, simply add more rope. Loop the center point of the folded new rope through an existing rope, then run the ends through the loop (a knot often called a "lark's head"). In many positions there will be one focal point where most of the rope is tied on to the bondage. In this position, it's just above the wrists in the middle of the upper back.

19. *"carefully resting on her clit hood just behind the pelvic bone"*

The crotch knot adds a great deal of sexual excitement to the scene for both men and women, but the positioning is very important. With women you have the option of placing the knot on the anus, the perineum, the vulva, or on or near the clitoris. This placement will be up to the sensual preference of the woman. A general suggestion, however, is to avoid placing it directly on the pelvic bone at the pelvic mound just in front of the clitoris. This tends to cause an uncomfortable bruising sensation for most women.

For men you have the option of placing the knot on the anus, perineum or just under the testes. You may also want to place one just above the upper base of the penis. This will form a rope cock-ring integral to the body harness that will heighten the self-awareness and pleasure for him.

Whether male or female, listen to their feedback in positioning and be prepared to adjust as necessary.

20. *"Creating a series of firm diamond shapes on her body"*

It's important in any bondage, but especially rope bondage, that the restraints be uniformly firm on the body. At a basic level, if the tension is uneven it'll feel unbalanced to the bound. It will also cause the lines to shift and sag differently as time goes on, making it visually unappealing to everyone involved. This unevenness in the ropes will lead to some parts of the body being less effectively bound than other parts.

More importantly, though, uniformly firm bondage is safe bondage... and loose bondage can be just as dangerous as overly tight bondage. If a person should faint or loose their footing or balance, loose bondage might cause them to twist a limb or, worse yet, choke. Think of bondage like a seat belt: a correctly positioned and firm seatbelt can save a person in case of an accident, but an ill-placed and loose one may lead to strangulation in addition to the original accident. (As a petite person, I'm acutely aware of this!) If an accident happens, firm bondage will actually act like another pair of hands, holding the person in place while you correct the situation.

There was an incident where one of my submissives began to feel light-headed while in a standing bondage with his arms

raised and body harness attached to a pillar. Since I could rely on the harness to keep him steady, I was able to undo his arms quickly and give him water. He regained his equilibrium quickly and I was able to untie the body harness while he stood steadily, with no risk of keeling over. Had the ropes been loose, I would have had to steady his body as well as to take care of all the other concerns.

21. *"Popping in a couple of fresh batteries"*

Could you imagine the disappointment if this top was caught without fresh batteries in the middle of the scene? Taking the time to visualize the scene at the beginning and set a plan into action will allow you to make sure that all the equipment you need is ready and right for the job. Check to see that any external structure you will rely on for support can safely take the strain and weight that might be placed on it and more. Make certain that you have the quantity and types of rope that you need for your scene. Make sure that you have the safety shears and any emergency items you might need. Of course, any battery-operated devices should never be stored with the batteries in place, so take the time to have fresh batteries on hand.

22. *"slide the vibe just above the knot at her rib"*

Another benefit of the uniformly firm rope harness is in its ability to conduct vibration throughout. Sliding the vibrator between the ropes will cause the entire harness to vibrate around the body of the submissive, bringing sensual awareness to the entire body and not just to the genitalia. This sensation is both surprising and delightful for the bottom and a pleasure to watch for the top. If the rope bondage is combined with intercourse, then both partners become direct beneficiaries of the sensual vibrations.

Slim vibrators work best for this, as they won't create a bulky, uncomfortable pressure point. Battery-operated ones give the freedom of mobility. In order to make the vibrator stay in place, take two lines that are lying together on the body and twist them once or twice. Then slide the vibe into that twist. The torsion of the twisted line will keep it in place. This is one of the few occasions when you place twists in the line against the skin.

23. *"I'll savor my sweet captive's quivering for a while... and then...."*

Don't rush a scene. Take your time! It's a common mistake to try to do a whole lot quickly, especially for rope bondage. You aren't doing this for a stage performance, you're doing this for the two of you. Remember that the pleasure is in the total sensuality and awareness of each moment. There are times when you need to stop what you are doing and let the bottom sink into the pleasure of all that's happening to her. If you insist on rushing through the experience you will have robbed both of you of this pleasure.

For the Bottom:

It may seem that there are fewer points of concern discussed here for the bottom, but this doesn't mean that they are less important or she is free of any responsibility. While what she brings to the scene may not be technically detailed, it's just as

critical in making the experience sizzling hot or dull and disappointing.

1. *"I stand naked before him, aroused... ready for our adventure. I shed my clothes and worries of the day."*

Don't let the concerns of the day enter into your scene. The burdens of the day will only distract you from enjoying the magic and pleasure of the experience fully. Don't cheat yourself like that. It's also disrespectful to the top to not be fully present and participatory by letting yourself be distracted. Play should be the one place where you can let your troubles go.

Unfortunately this isn't always easy. As we discussed for the top, each person must discover how to best they find their own "head space" or mindset before entering into play. It helps to find something to do that's ritualistic and different from the ordinary to create boundaries between the everyday and the special occasion of play. Some find it helpful to slowly and purposefully disrobe. Others find comfort and release from worry through a collaring ritual with their dominant at the beginning of the scene.

Beyond the physical nakedness, many find it helpful to approach a scene as being emotionally naked to one's partner. Letting go of defenses and pretenses that one might have up to the rest of the world is not necessary with your partner. Allow yourself the relaxation and freedom of emotional transparency and sweet vulnerability under the loving protection of your partner.

2. *"she... stretches"*

As discussed above, stretching and physical preparedness for the scene is very important in preventing injury or unplanned derailing of the play momentum. It is the bottom's responsibility to keep herself in a state of fitness, health and well-being suitable for the scene. This is not to say that she must be an athlete to play. This simply means that she must be realistic and exercise common sense. Any physical limitations, whether permanent or temporary, must be disclosed and discussed in advance. She needs to be realistic about what her body can take. If there's a propensity to motion sickness, then suspension bondage would not be a wise choice, regardless of how sexy and desirable it may seem.

The bottom also needs to make special preparations for play itself. Here are some points to consider.

- Has she had enough rest going into the scene? Exhaustion not only robs the bottom of fully experiencing pleasure, but can lead to accidents.

- Has she had adequate food and water?

- Has she stretched before the scene?

- Has she gone to the bathroom?

- Has she considered her state of mind and health for that moment and shared that with her top?

3. "I yield to his desire so that my desires may be freed"

This is closely related to the discussion of letting go of the mundane worries in order to enjoy the scene fully. It's a rare occasion in this modern world to be able to can surrender fully with deep trust. It may be extremely difficult, but ultimately deeply satisfying ,to find freedom in surrendering to the moment under the guidance of love. If you find it difficult to do so for the whole scene, as it can be a very unfamiliar territory for many, breathe deeply and surrender for just short periods of a scene and enjoy yourself. Eventually these periods will get longer and the feeling will become a familiar one... even a desired and delightful one that you come to look forward to.

4. "my wrists turn freely to caress his taut, naked belly"

It is just as much her responsibility to give feedback beyond simple safewords, as it is the top's duty to monitor her condition throughout the scene. Pragmatically speaking, it's in the bottom's best interest to let the top know if something is working so he'll keep doing that, and conversely when something is not working so that he can stop doing whatever is counterproductive to pleasure or potentially injurious. This is not to say that she needs to be able to give full analytical verbal feedback at the drop of a hat. That would be counterproductive, as it would keep her in an analytical state rather than allowing her to surrender to the experience. Often the bottom, profoundly affected by the pleasure and magic of the rope experience, is not in the mood for, or even capable of, being verbal.

Therefore, feedback from the bottom may come in the most primal of expressions. Smiles, moans, head nodding, a grateful touch, elated giggling and even tears of joy are all appropriate feedback indicating that the experience is wonderful. Likewise, physical distress and emotional limits must be expressed. For this I really prefer if the bottom is able to clearly tell me what's going on. Safewords and direct words or pointing are much appreciated by the top. Every bottom expresses pleasure and dislike differently. The bottom should take the time to consider how they react to each of these and let the top know. The insightful top will take the time to ask this as well.

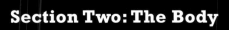

Section Two: The Body

Getting Started: Rope Selection & Safety

Selecting Your Rope

The ideal rope is one that you and your partner enjoy. Really, I'm not joshing you. Each rope bondage enthusiast has his or her personal favorites... I certainly have mine. I suggest that you try various different kinds and see which ones you like best. Different ropes have different properties and characteristics that may or may not work with your scene. It's good to have a general sense of what these are.

Here's a list of many different types of rope and rope-like materials that I've used or considered for scenes. This is certainly not an exhaustive list.

Cotton	Plastic tubing
Coir (coconut husk)	Bungee
Sisal	Sash cord
Manila	Strips of Kimono
Jute	Silk
Hemp	String of costume pearls
Nylon	Magician's rope
Polypropylene	Webbing
Polyester	Parachute cord
Rubber	etc…
Leather	

What other ideas for rope or rope-like materials do you have?

I know what some of you are thinking. You've seen those amazing photos of Japanese rope bondage with the kind of brown hemp rope we use on the cover of this book, and that surely that must be the authentic stuff. Yes, it is. But the Japanese rope masters who'll use the hemp rope are just as likely to use other materials as well to suit their personal preferences and experiential needs. I know one fellow who prefers cotton lines over hemp. There are also many photos where I have seen rubber, nylon and even chain used like rope. Having said this, I will be honest with you: my personal favorite is the softened hemp rope, which I'll discuss in more detail shortly.

Other considerations for selecting your rope may also include diameter, length, method of weave, texture, tensile strength, stretch, flex and color.

Sources for Rope

There are many places where you can obtain quality rope affordably, even in the most conservative, remote and non-kinky places. In addition, rope is generally much cheaper than equipment specifically made for erotic bondage play, adding to the versatile charm of rope bondage.

Here are some places where you can find rope that might appeal for your play. Make sure to ask fellow bondage enthusiasts in your area for their favorite local suppliers. As an enthusiast I'm always finding interesting sources and sharing them with my friends as well

Hardware store
Marine supply store
Mountaineering supply
Military surplus store
Fabric store
Magic supply store
Bondage and sex toy shops
The World Wide Web
Local and national leather events (they often have vending areas)

Texture and Material

Texture and material of the rope are major concerns for your *shibari* pleasures. Since most of the rope used in Japanese rope bondage will touch the body and skin directly, you'll want to carefully consider the feel of the rope against the skin and what effects you wish to create. While I'm not able to discuss all possible ropes, here are a few of the materials to consider…

Cotton rope is very soft and gentle on the skin. It'll soften with usage and washing to the skin's delight. When it's new it tends to have a good deal of flex and give, making it an excellent rope for the novice bottom. It may be comforting for some of them to feel the rope give and stretch to their breathing. Cotton rope dyes well, so you can custom color your own rope. Cotton also has a "high burn speed," meaning that the rope has to run along the skin much faster before it'll create a blister. Thus it's much

kinder on the skin than other ropes such as nylon or polypropylene. Another advantage is that cotton rope holds knots better than many other materials. I find the magician's rope (available in magic and novelty stores) wonderfully soft and nicely sized for bondage. On the other hand, cotton lines are generally not made for heavy-duty work or rated for load bearing. Depending on the construction, cotton rope may also have been woven inconsistently, leading to possible breakage under stress. It also has a lot of stretch in it. Keep these issues in mind if you are considering supporting a significant portion of a bottom's weight.

Nylon seems to be one of the most popular ropes used for bondage in America today, as it's widely and cheaply available in many sizes and colors. It's smooth, soft and silky on the skin. Nylon does stretch (although not as much as cotton), so it's another rope that's kind to the body in that way. On the other hand, it does have a lower burn-speed, possibly causing burns and abrasions sooner than cotton, so you'll want to be careful as you run the line across the body. Nylon doesn't dye as easily as cotton, so it'll be worth getting the ropes pre-colored if you are fashion-conscious. Imagine, a scene where the ropes on the submissive matches the color of one's latex gown! (Not that I'd ever do such a thing, mind you!) One of the down sides of nylon is that due to its silkiness it does not hold a knot as well or as tightly as some natural fibers such as cotton and hemp.

Climbing rope may seem like an unusual suggestion, but if you want to make sure that there's full support for supporting the submissive to an external frame, there's no doubt that climbing rope will meet your tensile strength needs. It's rough on the skin, not soft nor really flexible, and can burn on the skin quickly, so it's not a rope that's suited for ties on the body.

Hemp ropes: The most traditional of the Japanese bondage ropes is the twisted hemp or hemp-jute blend rope. It's a beautiful golden color when new and then over time and loving use seasons to a darker ash-brown. Once properly treated, hemp is soft and sensual to the skin with a most pleasing and unique scent reminiscent of cut grass or hay. As discussed earlier, I like to associate this scent with bondage pleasure in the heart and minds of my play partners. It has a very high burn speed, so you're less likely to burn the skin as quickly as you would with nylon. It also holds knots and ties extremely well. This is the rope that is most often seen with and identified with Japanese style rope bondage. It's probably the closest to what was historically used in medieval *Hojo-jutsu*. It is difficult to obtain authentic Japanese hemp rope, pre-treated and ready for the binding arts, without contacts in Japan, but we can use our own resources and make our own.

With some searching you can locate twisted hemp rope domestically produced as well as from overseas. It will look like a thick version of twine. When you first get it, you'll first notice how rough and scratchy the texture is. You'll wonder what on earth you're doing putting this on the delicate skin of your loved ones. Please remember that the rope you have in this condition has not been prepared for bondage use. Right now it's suitable for binding trees in Japanese ornamental gardening and tree branch forming – but certainly not pleasant for people!

To prepare hemp for softness suitable to use on people, here's what I do: Cut the hemp to your desired length. (Length suggestions are discussed below.) Tie off the ends in an overhand knot to prevent them from fraying. Boil a very large stockpot full of water and cook the rope in it for a while – maybe an hour or so – while frequently stirring with a wooden spoon. Add water if the level lowers significantly. Drape the hemp in large, loose loops over a clothesline to dry. Let it dry fully – in a high humidity area, like here in San Francisco, it might take a day or two. Check to see if the rope is considerably softer. It does not have to be at your ideal softness at this time, as the next few steps will continue to soften it.

The next part takes a bit of care and attention to keep from burning your rope, your fingers, or, worse still, your whole house. Set up a candle or some other small fire source such as a chemistry alcohol burner on a stable surface. Remove any fire hazards and have some water or fire extinguisher nearby. Light the fire. Take the end of the rope and using a slow rotating motion, carefully singe off the "split ends" or the rough frays from the length of rope. This is a painstaking process, so don't rush it.

Once the rough strands are burned off and shaken out, then carefully massage in small dabs of oil into the rope. Just a bit on your hand will do nicely. I tend to like mink oil but I've also heard of others using plain petroleum jelly. Massage it in until the oil is fully absorbed. Let the rope hang dry loosely for a few days to let the rope "age" into the new condition.

Ends of the Rope

There are many ways to finish the ends of most rope to keep it from fraying. For natural fibers such as hemp and cotton, I personally prefer a simple overhand knot at the ends, as I mentioned earlier. It's just my preference for a more rustic look. Whipping the ends, where a smaller thread or twine is wrapped or stitched around the ends, is also very attractive, if labor-intensive. If you have a dominant/submissive relationship with a service component, it might be quite appropriate for the submissive to prepare the ropes in which he'll be bound. Some simply wrap electrical tape on the ends. Others dip the ends in a can of liquid latex, available in hardware stores, often called "tool handle dip" or "tool dip."

A quick way to finish the ends of synthetic rope is to quickly expose it to flame and let the ends lightly melt. Be careful with this method, as liquefied nylon and other synthetics are extremely hot and can cause a terrible burn on skin, carpet, floors, etc., and the fumes are not too pleasant either. Burning the ends of synthetic rope is quick but it can also create uneven sharp ends that can scratch skin unpleasantly. Of course you can't use this last method with natural fiber rope, as it'll simply catch fire.

Another option is to not finish the ends at all. If the rope is woven, not twisted, it will unravel up to a certain point and then just stop fraying. As the rope runs over the skin and under other lines, there will be no foreign material or unevenness on the skin, just softness. The soft whip-like ends may also be used for sensation play.

Size

Length: There's no absolute length that the rope must be. The rope must be manageable and practical to suit your purpose. The length commonly used by the Japanese rope masters to bind female models has been 7 meters, or approximately 21 feet, but I've heard that they've been lengthening that due to increase in the average size of the Japanese woman. Cut the rope to approximately 7 to 8 meter lengths. That's approximately 21 to 25 feet. Due to the larger average stature of Westerners, I would suggest the 25-foot length – much longer than that and it becomes difficult to manage. Most of the poses in this book are based on one or more 25-foot lengths.

Diameter: Rope diameter of practical bondage usage generally ranges from 1/8 inch (approx. 3mm) to 3/4 inch (approx. 20 mm). Many of the hemp ropes in Japan range from 6mm to 8mm (approx. 1/3 inch).

Generally speaking, the medium ropes are better suited for torso harnesses, limbs and binding to external structures such as chairs and poles. Thicker ropes are great for suspension support lines and load-bearing lines. Thinner ropes are wonderful for decorative work, CBT (cock and ball torment), hands, feet and some types of head bondage. The thinner the rope is, the more it will cut into the person when pressure is applied. This could lead to lost circulation or nerve damage.

If you anticipate such a pressure you have a few choices. First, you can simply use rope with a larger diameter. This spreads out the pressure to a wider area, distributing the force and reducing risk considerably. Or you can wrap smaller-diameter rope on the area several times, effectively increasing the contact area between the rope and skin, again redistributing the pressure.

Rope Care and Maintenance

Keep your ropes well cared for. The rope will be touching the skin of someone you care about. Respect your play partner, the rope and the spirit of the play by taking good care of your ropes. For the same reason my bondage ropes do not cross over to utilitarian non-bondage purposes.

Storing rope: To keep your play rope separate from utility ropes create a specific place where they are kept. This might be a duffel bag, a box, a particular shelf, or your dedicated playroom or dungeon. Store clean ropes only and set aside soiled rope for cleaning. The ropes should not be stored in a damp place or stored wet, as you don't want your lines to get mildewed.

If you don't use your ropes frequently, store them loosely coiled to prevent them from getting "bad habits." If you use them frequently, store them coiled in a way that they're ready for use. The sight of a dominant fumbling with her rope at the beginning of a scene is hardly submission-inspiring. Style is, after all, such an important part of Japanese rope play!

Since most of the ties start with the center-point of the doubled line, it's easiest to have that be the first thing that you untie on the skein. To store it this way, start by folding the line in two and grasping the ends of the rope evenly in one hand. Then wind the doubled rope from the hand to elbow, leaving a yard length of doubled line free. Take the wound line off your arm. Coil the loose yard of doubled line around the wound-up body of the rope, then simply tuck the last bit, the center loop, under the last wrap so just the very end sticks out. This last loop showing will always be the center point. When the time comes to play, all you need to do is to reach to your rope, grasp it by the center point and unfurl it with great gusto!

Cleaning rope: Rope gets dirty from hot play. That's just a reality. Like intimate clothing it absorbs the sweat, tears, desire and all sorts of body fluids... and eventually the time comes to wash it. If you play out of doors it might also pick up materials from your environment.

Excessive washing of your rope will cause it to break down quickly, so use your common sense about when to wash. If you only play with one partner, you may be washing less frequently than if you have multiple play partners. If your bondage is done over clothing the ropes will require less washing than those used against flesh. Levels of exposure to sex fluids, blood, saliva and other body fluids will also determine your washing frequency.

As mentioned earlier, set aside the soiled ropes instead of putting them away with the clean ones. To make things easier after play I suggest that you tie your soiled ropes differently than you do your clean ones. I tie my soiled lines in a daisy-chain loop. This way they're ready to be washed. You may just want to have a designated dirty rope bag as well.

Hand washing your rope is an option but not one many like to take. Machine washing at a gentle cycle is fine. Use a large mesh "lingerie bag" to put the ropes in and you'll save yourself de-tangling time. Looping the rope in a loose daisy chain for the wash will also keep the rope controlled during the wash cycle.

Use a mild detergent, preferably something that's scent- and allergen-free. Avoid fabric softener, as many people are sensitive to it. I also feel that the scent of fabric softener will ruin the natural hemp fragrance.

If body fluid is a concern you will need to decide whether you want to add a bleach cycle or simply throw that rope away. Sometimes it's much safer to just throw away rope than to play guessing games with pathogens and your partners' health.

Line dry the ropes in large loops. Large loops will keep it from drying in "bad habits" from a tight coil. Don't dry it in a dryer, as shrinkage may be uneven in the ropes and the heat may degrade the structural strength of the rope, or, worse still, melt some of the synthetic ones.

Other Tools and Equipment

Other than rope, there are a few things that you need and a few more things that might be nice to have.

Must have:

- Safety shears or EMT scissors: All-purpose scissors that cut through tough materials like thick rope. EMT scissors have a flattened and rounded bottom side to prevent the skin from being cut. You never know

when there might be an emergency and the rope must come off the bottom faster than you can say "Quick!"

- First aid kit: This is just common sense. Even something as simple as a little rope burn could use a bit of treatment and TLC.

- Water or other fluids to drink: As mentioned before, bondage is a physically demanding sport and the bottom can get quite thirsty quickly. If there's any open-mouthed breathing or gags in use, she will need water more frequently.

- CPR and First Aid certification: Again, common sense. Whether you play SM or not, whether you're in a dungeon or not, everyone should be trained in CPR and First Aid. You never know when you might be called upon to use it. For certification in your area just contact the American Red Cross at 800-520-5433. You don't need to explain why you might need it. After all, we are all concerned citizens!

Really nice to have:

- Marlinspike: A blunted spike used by nautical types for splicing rope. It's the best thing to break a tight knot without breaking your fingers. After all, I'd hate to break a nail!

- Blanket or coat: In all the excitement and exertion of bondage, sometimes the bottom suddenly gets cold. This could happen during or after play.

- Small towels: Great for padding between hard or uncomfortable parts. If the knees or ankles are bound together without padding, the area rubbing up against each other may become sore or bruised. If using external structures like dowels, chairs or frames, padding between that and the body may be nice. Also handy as a quick pillow or to wipe up any sweat or fluids. Truly a trick towel!

- Straw: So they can drink the water you kindly provided with some degree of comfort. This is one of those nice little touches that impress the bottom that you care. Of course, water delivered via a hot kiss is just as effective and so much sexier!

Might be fun to have:

- Block and tackle or pulley: Half the work and double the drama for partial or full suspension scenes. Take the time to set it up and figure it out before the scene. A winch with a ratchet to prevent the rope from sliding backwards is especially wonderful.

- Wooden dowel or bamboo pole: A very traditional Japanese touch: use the dowel or bamboo rod to bind your fantasy prisoner! Be sure that any rod you use is more than sturdy enough for its task – a pole breaking under a bottom's weight can cause a serious accident.

- Vibrator: See the discussion on vibrators on page 28.

- Camera: Only with everyone's consent! It's fun to enjoy your work of art after the scene... Don't make my past mistake of not having planned ahead... Oh, if only I had remembered a camera for all those great scenes...

- External bondage structures: The bed, a chair, a sturdy pillar, a tree, a table, a Saint Andrew's Cross, an overhead beam... you get the idea!

Safety Concerns

Perhaps this may sound alarmist to you. Perhaps you've heard the safety message so many times that you feel jaded. I'm sorry if you are. Safety concerns, however, are very real. In my early days of rope explorations as a bottom, I was in a rope bondage mishap that nearly crippled my left arm permanently. It was purely accidental and there is no one to blame except my own enthusiasm and masochistic machismo. I wasn't paying attention to the signals my body was sending me. I just ignored it so I could play greedily on. I am now grateful that this accident happened before I became a top, as I am now keenly aware of the potential for serious damage if you're not paying attention and if you don't know what you're doing.

So, I hope that you'll read on and brush up on your safety techniques. Here I'll discuss some of the highlights specifically relevant to rope bondage. For further in-depth discussion of safety concerns in bondage, please take the time to read *Jay Wiseman's Erotic Bondage Handbook* (Greenery Press, 2000).

Where to bind and where not to bind: Major muscle groups are wonderful to bind! Torso, upper arm, forearm, thighs and lower legs. With a bit of practice you can incorporate hands and feet. While the back of the neck can take a bit of pressure, as seen in the *Agura* position, the front of the neck should not have pressure on it as that can lead to choking, strangulation and blocked blood flow to the brain. With the exception of the hip joint we don't want to actually bind at the joints, as this may lead to injury of veins, arteries, lymph nodes, nerves, etc. What about wrist and ankle bondage, you ask? Ropes on wrists and ankles are actually applied to the leg or forearm just above the joint. While it might appear that the rope is on the joint itself, the pressure is actually primarily on the leg or forearm. A properly bound wrist/ankle restraint, not too tight, with plenty of play, will save these limbs in any scene from potential injury.

Never bind too tightly: While the rope needs to be on firmly, it should not be so tight as to cut off circulation or cut into nerves. Make sure that a finger can slide between the bound skin and the rope. If the ropes might be on too tightly adjust their position or loosen them a bit.

Has it tightened or loosened on its own? Rope bondage can tighten or loosen on its own. It may be due to the natural stretch in the rope, gradual contraction of the tissue under the rope, shifting of the bottom's body position, their straining against the rope, or tension from counter-directional rope. Periodically check as you bind as well as during the scene and make necessary adjustments.

External structures. So you decided to use external structures as we discussed above. Can the structure survive the passion of your scene? Before you play, apply the expected stress and force on it… and more. The last thing you want is the structure to come crashing down on you and your partner.

Cutting the rope. If there's an emergency, be willing to cut the rope with your EMT shears. Remember, your rope is cheap, your date may feel cheap, but trust is golden.

Having said that, with a little planning and a level head during moments of crisis, you'll reduce the probability of having to ever cut your rope. As discussed on page 24, visualizing and planning your scene in advance will help you identify potential weak points and problem areas that might develop into numb limbs or restricted breathing. If you see such points, then bind them in such a fashion so that these areas can be untied immediately. Sometimes a panicked situation is more psychological; a calming top can reduce the anxiety and buy time to slowly and safely bring the person to a sense and situation of safety. Remember: Don't panic.

Itchy rope? Some people might be mildly allergic to various natural fiber ropes such as hemp. Check for rashes. Wash the area and proceed with any allergy treatment that the person commonly uses or is prescribed.

Stretch! Read pages 23 and 30!

Rope burn? Rope marks? Treat them as you would other mild skin abrasions. Wash the area and apply ointment if necessary. (For more detailed first aid tips, see p. 156.) Healthy, moist and supple skin is less likely to get slight abrasions and scratches from rope. Remember, bottoms: moisturize!

Generally rope marks are simply pressure marks, like the marks from socks. They fade quickly.

Other health concerns? Make sure to fully discuss any health concerns before you play. Special issues to discuss might include circulatory problems, epilepsy and other seizure disorders, problems in any joint, back trouble, breathing problems, and heart trouble, as well as any history of bondage-related emotional trauma.

The Knots and Ties

Now, it's finally time to look at the ties and knots! Whenever I teach classes on rope bondage I see anxious faces worried that they don't know how to tie fancy knots. Please don't worry about all those fancy knots that you never bothered to learn in summer camp. If you can tie your shoelaces, you can do rope bondage!

I also like to remind people that being a rope bondage enthusiast doesn't mean that you have to be a knot fetishist. What's the difference? A knot fetishist enjoys making pretty knots whether there's someone in them or not. A rope bondage enthusiast is a person who comes up with creative ways to restrict a person's mobility by using rope. The latter's emphasis is on the interpersonal dynamics that the rope facilitates. I believe that it's more important to develop the sense of overall position and function of the bondage than to start with the focus on individual knots.

In fact, I'll share a secret with you. I don't know fancy knots. I just know some basics like the overhand, square knot, granny knot, bow knot and a few hitches and half hitches. I will do my best to describe to you the ties without complicated names (probably because I don't know them). If you need a refresher on these basics, or if you enjoy knowing fancy knots, I encourage you to pick up one of the many books on knots out there.

The methods of binding that we'll look at in the following section are each one of many variations on a theme. I've tried to pick the easiest ones. These basics will allow you to see patterns in other bondage and enable you to figure out how others did theirs differently. This will eventually lead you to developing your own style.

Section Three: The Techniques

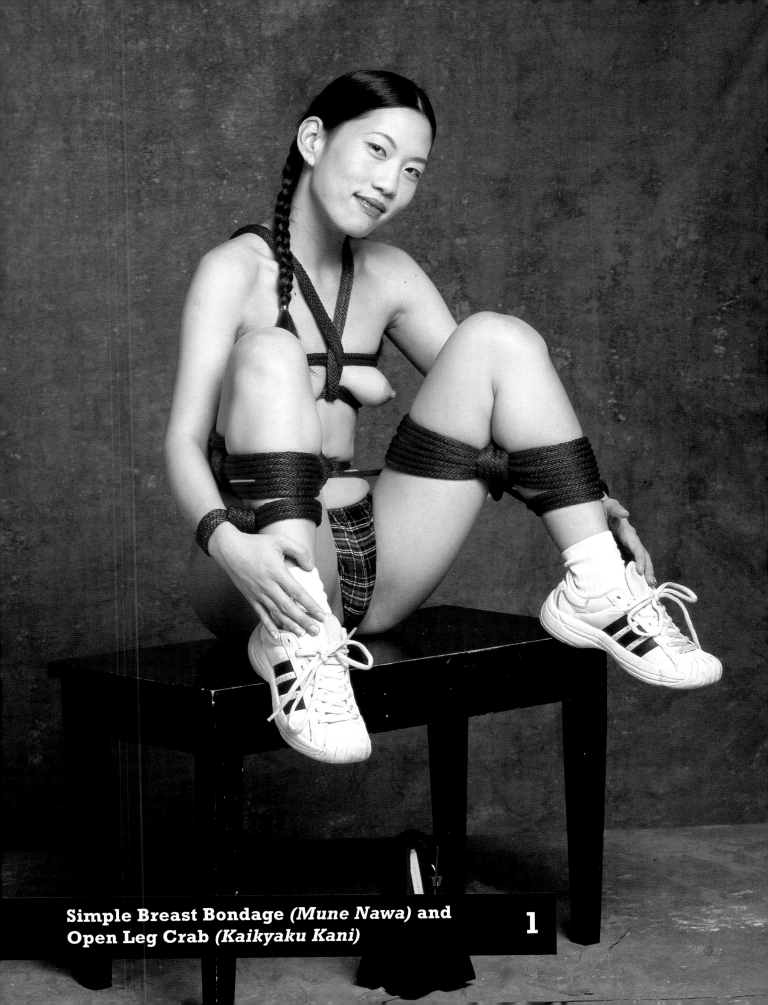

Simple Breast Bondage (Mune Nawa) and Open Leg Crab (Kaikyaku Kani)

1

Position 1:
Open Leg Crab *(Kaikyaku Kani)* and Simple Breast Bondage *(Mune Nawa)*

He moves my legs this way and that and the ropes fly again. Soon I'm tightly bound and spread open, the ropes digging deeper into my wet lips. My desire is so transparent to him... Self-consciousness rises under his gaze and my face burns in the flush of embarrassment of how exposed my eagerness for him is. Here and now he will not let me hide my wanton lust. Aroused even more by my own embarrassment, I can do nothing but present my body to his probing gaze. I wallow in my sweet helplessness... Although I'm not sure if I'm helpless now in his ropes or in facing my own desires.

This is an easy and enjoyable bondage for both the novice top and the novice bottom. Beyond its simple elegance, it's also one of the best rope bondage positions for sex: definitely in the "sexable" bondage category! I chose to show these two ties together, but they can be used independently or in combination with other ties.

Sexual accessibility and emotional vulnerability makes this position highly erotic and a favorite of many couples. The ropes on the breasts, with a bit of tightening, heighten sensual awareness for both men and women. The Open Leg Crab also allows for a fair amount of movement and change of position during play. Once bound, the bottom can be seated, placed on her back, or put on her knees with her face into the floor.

The Open Leg Crab is actually a very mobile bondage, comfortable for most body types, even for those with somewhat limited endurance, mobility or flexibility. You may choose to bind your bottom firmly to external structures to restrict movement further. The Open Leg Crab works delightfully in armchairs. If you do this on the bed, run a rope under the bed frame and attach it to the leg bondage, then pull the lines until the legs are opened firmly yet comfortably. You can also rig similar ropes from your bedposts for the same effect.

For a more traditionally Japanese scene with elements of erotic humiliation, the submissive would not be secured to an external frame, but would be moved, rolled and shoved around in bondage. This scene works well with a captive fantasy or sex slave scenario. Another traditional touch would be to place a bamboo rod at the crook of the leg, running from one leg to another and secured, forming a rustic spreader bar. Now the bottom may be rolled around and can squirm, but will not be able to close her legs.

Step by Step: Simple Breast Bondage *(Mune nawa)*

1.   Fold the rope in half. Place the center loop on the spine at about the same height as the center of the breasts.

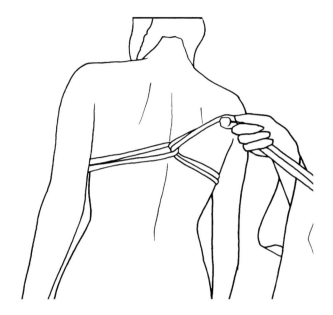

2.   Holding the center loop in place, wrap the doubled rope around the ribcage just under the breast. I suggest moving the sub around instead of moving yourself whenever possible. Make sure that the rope is on the ribcage and not under it. If the rope is under the ribcage, some subs may find that it interferes with breathing and comfort.

3. Bring the rope back around to the back.

4. Bring rope end through center loop and tighten the lines snugly around the ribcage.

5. Take the loose end of the rope and wrap it around the rib cage in the opposite direction, placing it above the breasts.

6. Bring the rope back around to the back.

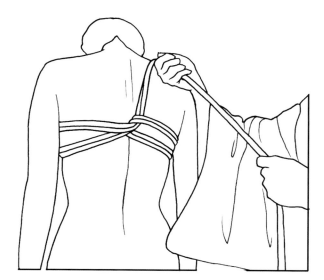

7. Loop the loose end of the rope through the last rope bend. Tighten the lines snugly around the ribcage. Here we only wrapped the ropes above and below the breasts once for simplicity, but you may wrap more if you wish. If there's going to be any serious weight or pressure placed on these chest lines I recommend wrapping a few more times to distribute the pressure.

8.   Bring the end of the rope up over the bottom's shoulder.

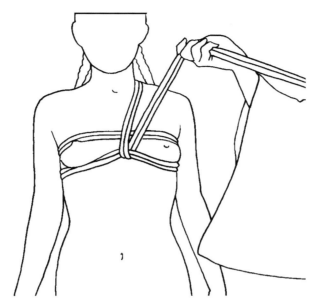

9.   Take the loose ends and run them over all the lines, then move under the ropes heading up. Hitch the ends under themselves.

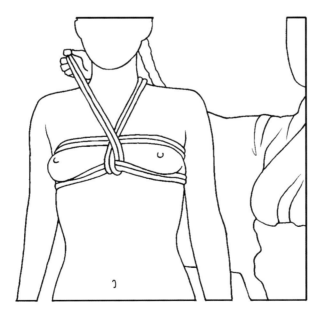

10. Continue the loose lines over the other shoulder.

11. Cross the ends over the lines coming down from the shoulders, and under the lines around the chest. A decisive tug will tighten the chest lines. This motion is psychologically dominant as well as serving to engorge the area with blood, thus increasing sensitivity. This is true for both men and women.

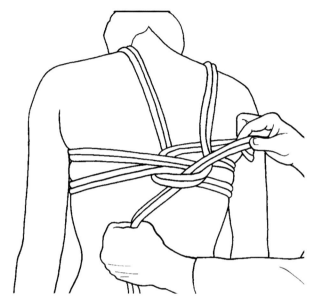

12. Return lines to the knot at the center of the spine and tie off with an overhand or square knot.

Options and Ideas: If you have excess rope at this time, you may choose to use it for further bondage. Here are some options.

    a. Use the lines to bind the wrists together at the center of the back.

    b. Bring the line down along the spine to waist level and begin a body harness. You can use the same technique as the Tortoise Shell *(Kikkou)*, simply starting it from the back to front.

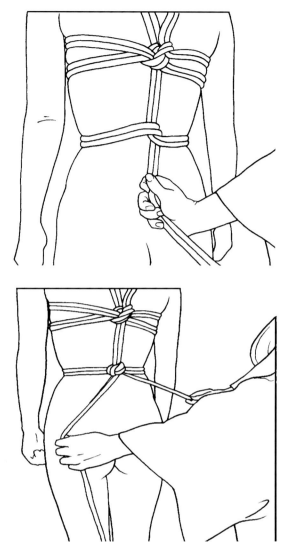

c. Use the lines to attach the chest harness to an external structure such as a pillar or chair back.

d. Create a "handle" on the back by coiling the loose ends tightly around the ropes on the back. Finish off with an overhand knot or a hitch.

Step by Step: Open Leg Crab
(Kaikyaku Kani)

I started the one in the photo with a waist rope purely as a personal preference, as I find waist ropes to be most practical: they provide another anchor point should I choose to further immobilize the bottom later on. The waist rope in itself is not part of the Open Leg Crab. Here I'll describe two ways to do this position, one with the waist rope and the other without.

Simple Open Leg Crab

1.   Fold the rope in half.

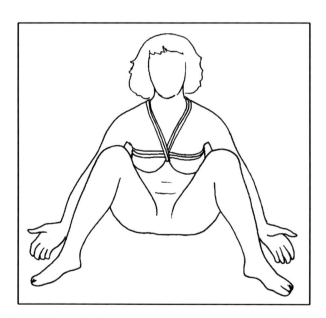

2.   Place the bottom on her rear or on her back with their legs bent to their chest. Place the wrists at corresponding ankles. This may be either inside the legs or outside the legs.

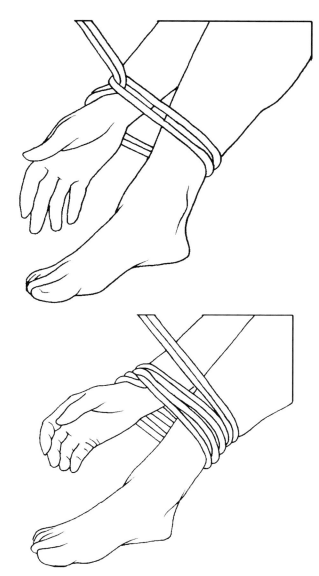

3. Place the center loop of the rope at the wrist, and thread the ends through it. Wrap the rope around wrist and ankle a few times. Make sure there's a gap of an inch or so between the ankle and wrist. This slack will be taken up in a moment.

4. Pass the loose end over the all ropes between the ankle and wrist. Bring the ropes forward again from under the wrapped rope. Now with a tug you can take up the slack between the ankle and wrist. Don't bind this too tightly. Make sure the wrist can move freely.

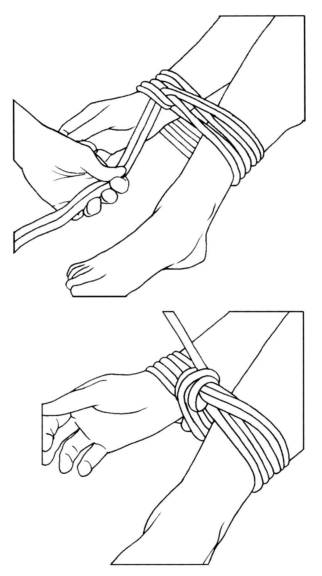

5. Tie off the rope with a hitch or overhand knot, securing the wrist tie.

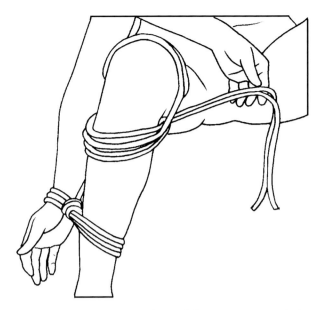

6. Wrap the remainder of the rope around the thigh and shin a few times.

7. In the same way you tied off the horizontal lines on the wrist to ankle, tie off the lines between the thigh and shin. Finish with a hitch.

Open Leg Crab With a Variation... Starting From a Waist Rope

1. Fold the rope in half.

2. Place the center loop on the stomach at about waist level.

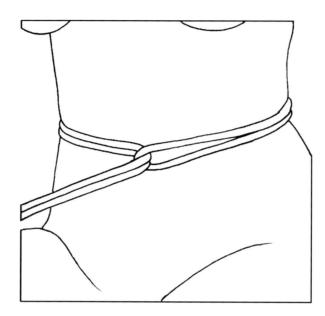

3. Holding the center loop in place, wrap the doubled rope around the waist. This line needs to be snug but not tight.

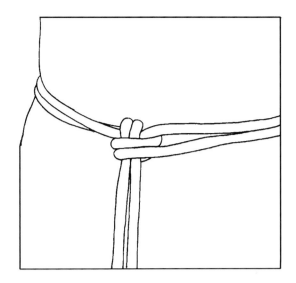

4.   Bring the rope back around to the front.

5.   Bring rope end through center loop and tie it off with a hitch.

6.   Separate the two ropes. One goes to the right and the other to the left leg.

7. Place the bottom on her rear or on her back with her legs bent to her chest, as close to the chest as possible. Wrap one of the free ropes around the thigh and shin a few times.

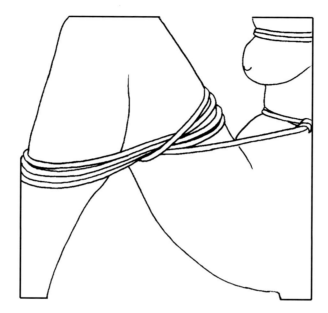

8. At the final wrap, bring the loose end across the entire band, cross it over the first wrap and pass it between the thigh and shin.

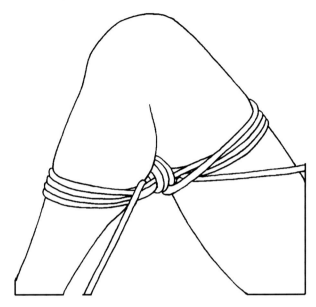

9. Bring it back under the band to its starting point. Tie it off with a hitch.

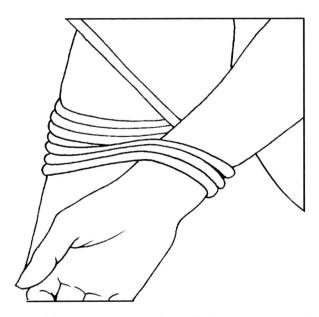

10. Take the remainder of the rope, move it down and wrap it around the wrist and ankle a few times. Make sure there's a gap of an inch or so between the ankle and wrist. This slack will be taken up in a moment.

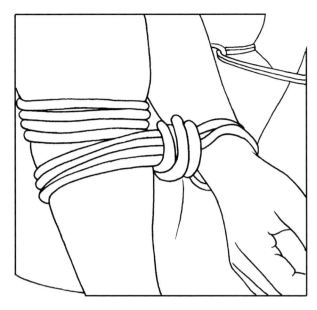

11. In the same way you tied off the horizontal lines on the thigh to shin, tie off lines between the wrist and ankle. Finish with a hitch. Here I suggest at least a double half hitch to prevent the wrist restraint from tightening down further. Make sure that there's enough room for the wrist to move freely.

Options and Ideas: These options can be used with either variation on the crab leg bondage if you have extra rope after you're finished.

    a. Tie it off to an external structure such as the sides of the bed, bedpost, chair back or arms.

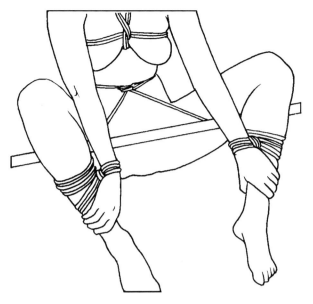

b. Slide a dowel or bamboo rod into the crook of the legs and use the excess rope to secure it, thereby forming a spreader bar.

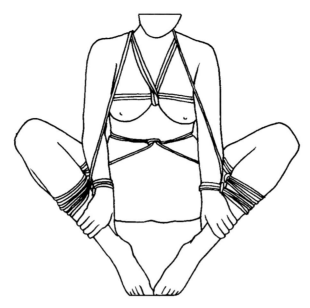

c. Run the excess rope from one leg around the back of the neck and to the other leg. Tie it off. Do the same with the other leg. This forms a "sling" for the legs, forcing them open without the obstruction of the pole. Placing a towel between the neck and rope is a kind touch.

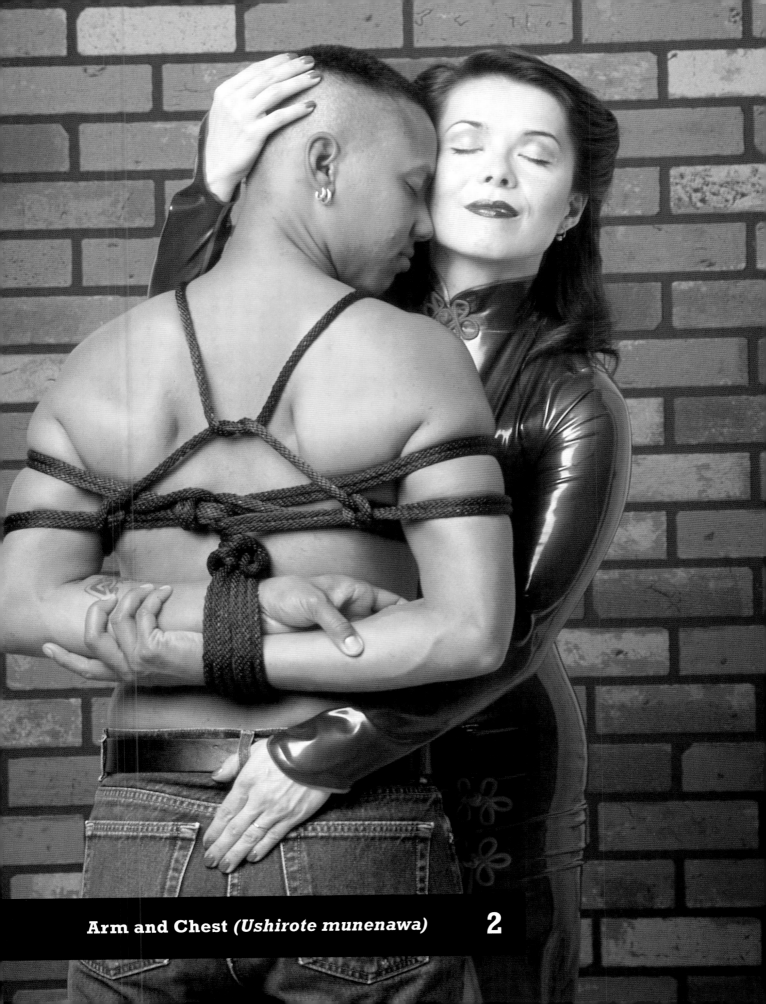

Arm and Chest (Ushirote munenawa)   **2**

Position 2:
Arm and Chest *(Ushirote munenawa)*

She stands behind me, pressing her beautiful body into mine as she seduces me with her voice. My sex starts to throb and swell. Soft hands run along my arms as I relax into her touch. Her hands rest at my wrists and she slowly brings them back, crossing them between us. I can feel the heat of her sex just beyond my fingers. I behave, remembering that a submissive must not take liberties. Keeping my wrists in one hand she reaches over to the pile of jewel-colored ropes, selecting one of deep ruby and unfurling it in a cascade of color. Swiftly my wrists are bound behind my back, and then my arms and torso soon follow in their fate of immobility. As the ropes tighten I can feel my nipples harden. Another rope flies up to the ceiling and she loops it through a bolt. A quick tug and I'm forced up onto my toes, carefully balanced. I am now at her mercy.

The *Ushirote munenawa* is one of the classic prisoner bondage techniques. It allowed the captive to be forced to move by his own locomotion, but the arm restrictions considerably hampered his speed and mobility.

As you'll see, this basic tie is the foundation for many other positions. It can be combined with other ties to create physically severe positions such as the hog-tie *(Gyakuebi)* and the cross-legged *(Agura)*. These "endurance" or "suffering" positions were used during interrogations. This basic arm tie can also be used to form other nicer, more "sexable" positions as well. It's a lot of fun when combined with the Open Leg Crab position. Depending on the size of the bottom, you may want a 35-foot or even a 50-foot rope for this position.

I caution you to be watchful of the arms and hands in this position. It's easy to get overly enthusiastic and tie the arm restraints too tight, leading to loss of circulation or nerve pressure down the arm. Pay attention to the temperature of the hand. Occasionally have the bottom grasp your hand. That way you can be sure of skin temperature as well as responsiveness and mobility. Make sure the bottom understands her responsibility to give you feedback in play.

Step by Step: Arm and Chest
(Ushirote munenawa)

1. Fold the rope in half. Bring the wrists together behind the bottom's back.

2. Wrap the wrists with the rope a few times forming a band, leaving the center loop hanging about 8 to 10 inches from the wrists. Make sure there's a gap of an inch or so between the wrists. This slack will be taken up in a moment.

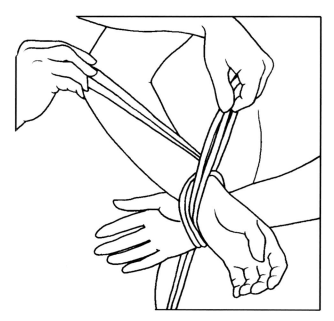

3. Cross the end with the center loop over the other free hanging ropes.

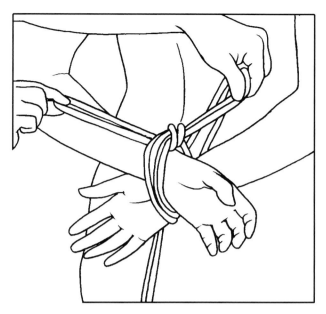

4.   Wrap the line with the center loop around the wristband, cinching the band together between the wrists. Wrap as often as you need to take up the slack, but make sure that the wrists can move freely to prevent possible injury.

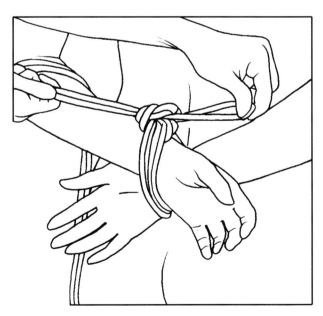

5.   With the loop and the other free ropes make a simple overhand knot, square knot or granny knot.

6. You should be left with an inch or two of the loop end showing and most of the free ends hanging loose. This tie is your wrist quick release. Should the arms lose circulation or get tingly, you can effortlessly untie the wrists. Sometimes just untying the wrists and dropping the arms will help the body recover, thus no further rope adjustments may be necessary. Then you may choose to simply tie the now loose wrists or forearms to the side of the body.

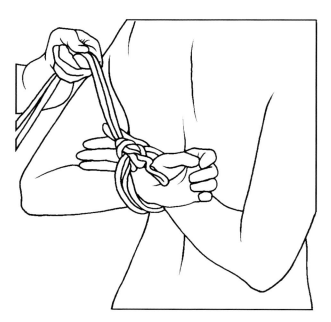

7. Tug on the free ends enough to move the wrists up the back to a desired position. The position of the wrists will depend on the bottom's flexibility.

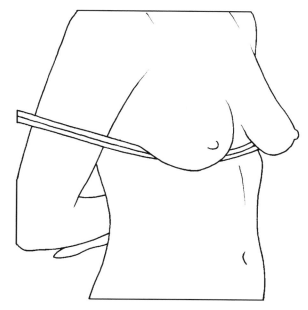

8. Wrap the doubled rope around the upper arms and rib cage just under the breast. I suggest moving the sub around instead of moving yourself whenever possible. Make sure that the rope is on the ribcage and not under it. If the rope is under the ribcage it may interfere with breathing and comfort. Bring the rope back around to the back over the biceps.

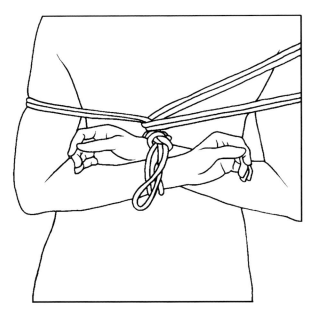

9. Bring the rope end through the center loop and tighten it snugly around the ribcage.

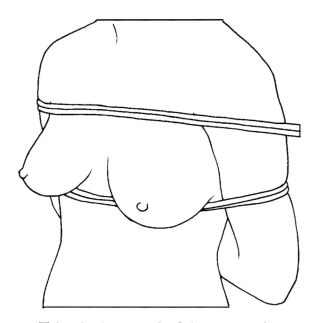

10. Take the loose end of the rope and wrap it around the upper arms and rib cage in the opposite direction, placing it above the breast. Bring the rope back around to the back over the biceps.

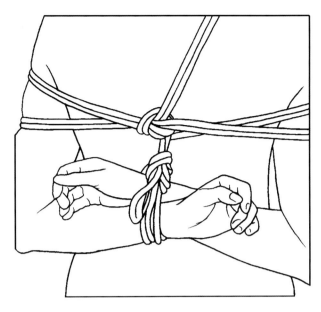

11. Loop the loose end of the rope through the last rope bend. Tighten the lines snugly around the upper torso. Here we only wrapped the ropes above and below the breasts once for simplicity, but you may wrap more if you wish. If there's going to be any serious weight placed on these chest lines I recommend wrapping a few more times to distribute the pressure. (You will, of course, need more rope if you wish to make these additional wraps.)

12. Take the loose ends, hook them over all the lines from the bottom, then move them under the ropes heading up. Hitch the rope under itself.

13. Now split the two lines. One will go right and the other left.

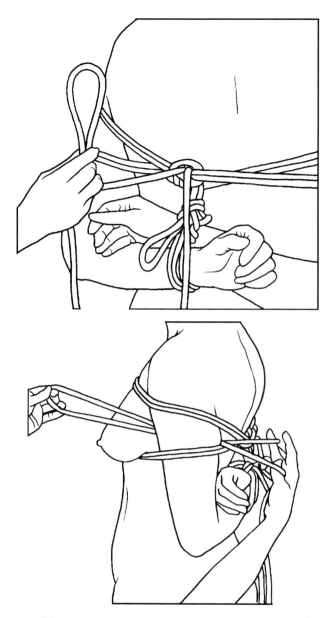

14. Take one line and move it to the right side. Fold a loop into the line. Move that loop between the upper arm and the torso, between the horizontal lines above and below the breasts. Pull the loop through but not completely, leaving the end on the back side.

17. Move the loop under the under-breast hori-zontal lines. Now the head of the loop should be sticking out towards the submissive's back.

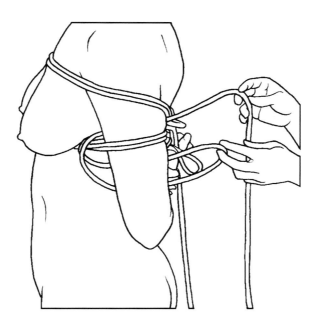

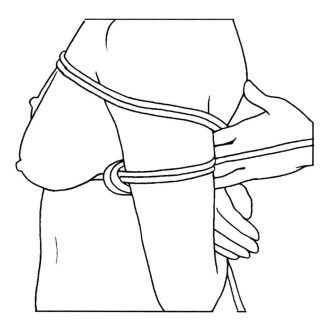

18. Take the end of the rope, which should still be hanging on the back from above the under-breast horizontal lines, and slide it through the loop sticking out. Slowly pull on that end rope. This should tighten down the loop across the horizontal lines.

19. Do the same on the other side.

20. Bring the two free lines together and do a simple overhand knot. If you run out of rope at this point, tie off the lines with a square knot. Add a second skein of rope by looping the center point around the knots at the center of the horizontal lines.

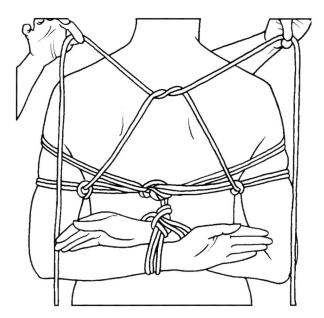

21. Separate the lines and move one over each shoulder to the front.

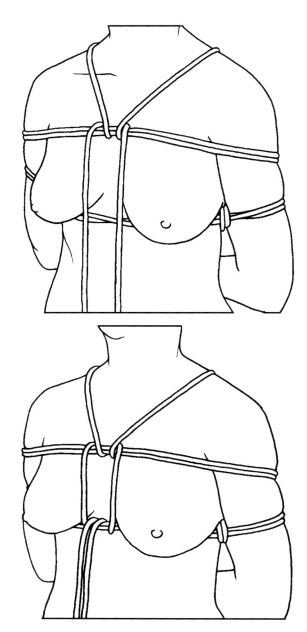

22. In a mirror-image symmetrical fashion, take both lines and hitch them over the upper breast lines. Do the same with the lower breast lines. A neat box shape should form between the two horizontal and two vertical lines.

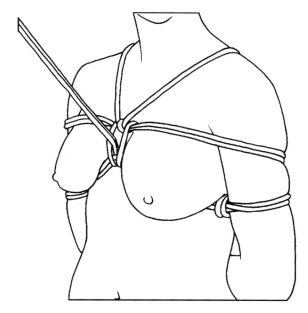

23. Here a decisive tug will tighten the breast lines. This motion is both psychologically dominant as well as serving to engorge the area with blood, thus increasing sensitivity. This is true for both men and women.

Options and ideas: At this point, the basic *Ushirote munenawa* is done. You may have free-flowing rope remaining. You may choose to do several things with the remaining rope.

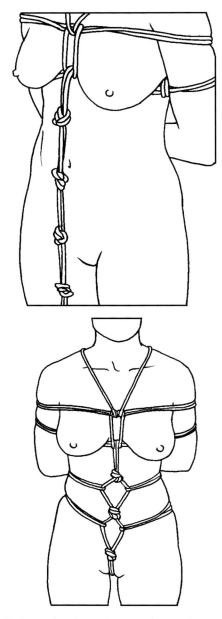

- Bring the line down along the stomach to begin a body harness. You can use the technique taught in the Tortoise Shell position.

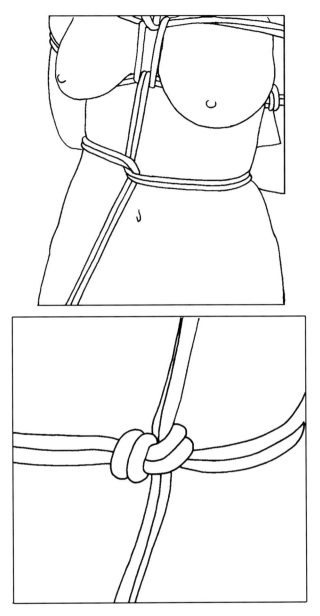

- Bring the lines down the stomach, wrap them around the waist and return to the front. Then tie the rope off to itself with a hitch to create a waist rope.

- Use the free end as a leash to move the submissive around with.

- Use this as the base for a Hog Tie (*Gyakuebi*).

- Combine with the Open Leg Crab *(Kaikyaku kani)* for a sexable position.

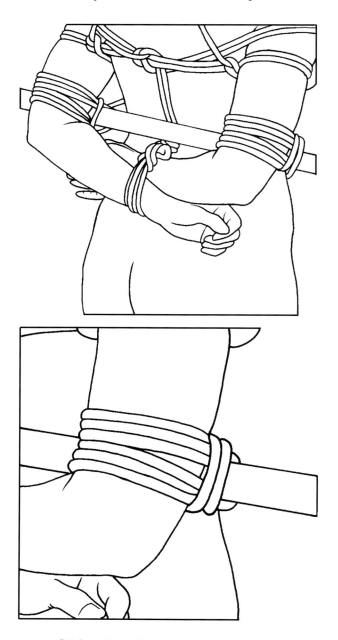

- Slide a dowel or bamboo rod in the crook of the arm behind the back for greater restriction. This also pushes the body and chest forward, heightening self-awareness.

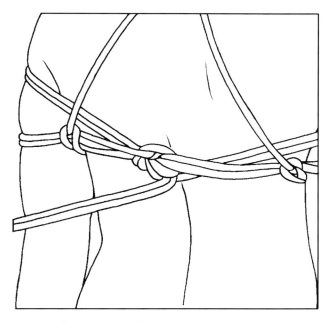

- Attach an additional rope to the knots at the center of the back. Connect that through a load-bearing point overhead. (Please refer back to the chapter on "Rope Selection and Safety" for more information on setting up safe load-bearing points.) Slowly pull that person up onto their toes. This is a very physically and psychologically vulnerable position borrowed directly from medieval interrogation. It's a great situation to do male genital play as he is fully exposed!

- From this tiptoe position, and with secure load-bearing ropes, you can bring up one leg for a classical Japanese asymmetrical form (explained later in Position 6, Crotch Harness and Partial Suspension).

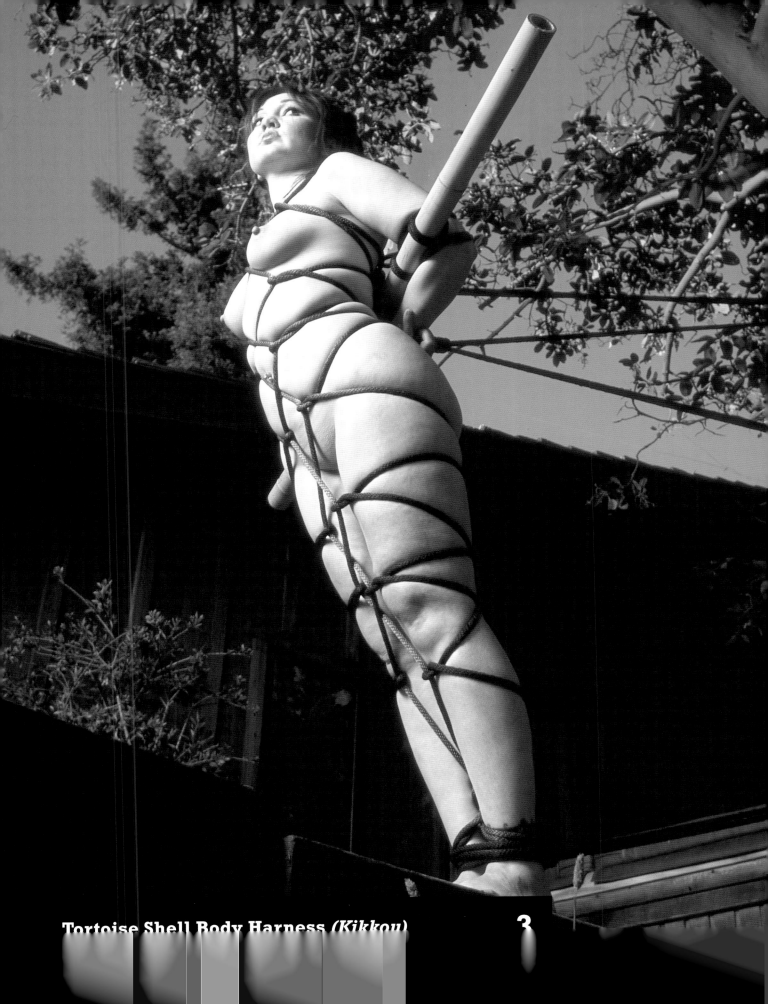

Tortoise Shell Body Harness *(Kikkou)*

3

Position 3:
Tortoise Shell Body Harness *(Kikkou)*

My nipples begin to tighten… part from the thrill of a new adventure, part from being a bit scared. Tonight she's going to take me on a new adventure… a longtime fantasy of mine. I want her to tie me up and be ravished by her love and adoration. She's so good to me and I trust her so much that I can finally try this.

With a sweet kiss she soothes my fears away. With loving firmness she caresses the curves of my body, eventually discovering my arousal. Gently she drapes the rope on my shoulders, letting it trail down to the curve of my belly. Then the rope slides between my legs, giving me a sweet shiver up by back. Swiftly she spins her web around me. My hands are free and she lets me caress her nakedness. I hold her voluptuous hips to assure myself that I'm not going to fly away from the lightheadedness of this new pleasure.

The *Kikkou* means "the tortoise shell" for its visually striking diamond pattern. Also known as the *Hishigata* ("diamond"), it's a beautiful ornamental body harness that's easy on the eyes and easier still on the body. Unless combined with other elements of shibari, it's not heavily constricting or physically challenging. Even with this less-than-restrictive quality, in the Japanese public's mind it has come to be recognized as a quintessential shibari form.

The *Kikkou* probably has its origin in the commoner's theater of the Edo period, rather than the secretive sects of martial artists practicing Hojojutsu. The general public may have become aware of it in the Kabuki theater, where it was used for its dramatic appearance and visibility even from the farthest seats. Compared to the practical *Ushirote munenawa* or the very restrictive *Agura* positions, this was a more theatrically appealing style in which colorful villains could be paraded bound, and captive female forms could be enhanced even over the kimono.

If the tortoise shell harness is simply an ornamental bondage that's not restrictive, why do I bother to teach it to you? Because, like so many things beautiful in Japan, it has its purpose – sometimes obvious and sometimes less so.

In its simplest form the Kikkou may appear to be just pretty rope on the body, leaving the bottom total freedom of movement. Under certain circumstances, however, this has its advantages. There are people who are interested in being bound in their sensual pursuits, yet at the same time find themselves nervous or apprehensive about bondage. For these people taking them directly to the more elaborate, restrictive and difficult positions may be too intimidating. They might be needlessly scared away from potential pleasure by experiencing too much too soon. For these people, I have found a gentler introduction to *shibari* by way of a pretty body harness to be just what the sex doctor ordered.

Initial exposure to rope bondage with a simple body harness allows the person to become accustomed to the feeling of rope on their skin and associate it with sensual self-awareness. For many, the feeling of a body harness simultaneously enhances a sense of sexy nakedness yet feel assuredly covered. There are others that enjoy the feel of the rope on the skin as a constant reminder of their lover's caress and intent.

I will let the novice rope bottom enjoy the body harness for a while, letting him become familiar with the pleasures before moving on to the next level. That may be during the same scene, or I may save the opportunity for a future play date. In either case, the body harness can be left on and used in the next level of play.

The other advantage of the rope body harness is its convenience in creating handles and anchor points for more restrictive or complicated positions. Many erotic bondage enthusiasts lament that the human form does not come with many original-issue bondage-friendly tie points. For many, this seems to limit them to the age-old four-point spreadeagle position. As visually appealing as this may be in fantasy, in reality the spreadeagle is not too restrictive and can be hard on the limbs.

By starting with a nicely tied rope body harness, however, you suddenly have many points and handles by which you can secure the bottom snugly to many different types of surfaces and other body parts. We'll look at some options in greater detail in the "Options and Ideas" section below.

I have seen many beautiful and different ways to tie the *Kikkou*. Here we'll discuss two of the simplest ways with a few variations. After you get the hang of these, you'll be ready for more variations as well as infusion of your own artistic touches!

Step by Step: The Knotted Tortoise Shell Body Harness (Kikkou)

1. Fold the rope in half.

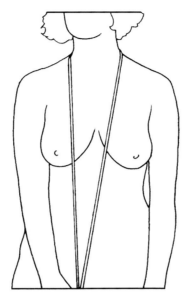

2. Place the center point on the spine at the back of the neck with the rest of the rope over the shoulders and breasts.

3. Bring the two lines together.

4. Tie a simple overhand knot at the sternum (chest bone). Avoid tying it closer to the neck than this, as you want to leave enough clearance around the neck for safety and comfort.

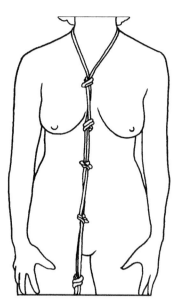

5. Place several overhand knots down the front of the body. This will look like a string of pearls. Let's call the knots "pearls" for shorthand. Depending on the appearance that you wish to create and the body type of the bottom, you may choose to do as few as two pearls or as many as... well, as many as you think attractive and practical in the binding. Three to four seems pretty typical. I tend to like to place the last pearl on the front of the torso just above the pubic bone for women and just at the upper base of the penis for men. My experience is that these are most sensual for the bound.

6. Bring the two lines between the legs to back of the body. Whether you place a crotch knot at this point or not is up to you. See the section on crotch knots on page 27 for further discussion on this question.

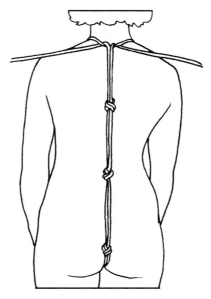

7. Repeat this process of creating a "string of pearls" with knots up along the spine. Take care not to place a knot on the tailbone, as this kind of pressure may be quite uncomfortable in a less-than-sexy way.

8. Take the two lines and pass the ends through the center point of the rope that rests at the back of the neck.

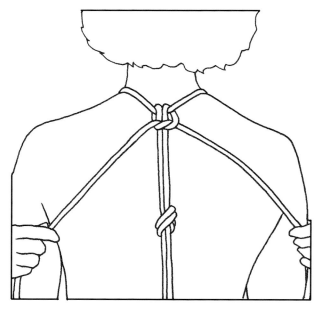

9. Separate the lines to the right and left sides and bring them over the rope on the spine. Tie them together with one overhand knot.

10. At this point this vertical ropes running up and down the body should be a bit on the loose side. As the bondage continues, the horizontal lines will take up the slack considerably. If this vertical foundation is too tight, further binding might be too uncomfortable for the bottom's pleasure or endurance. It's also difficult to create a visually appealing series of diamonds if there's no slack in the vertical lines.

11. Separate the lines again and bring them under each arm to the front of the body.

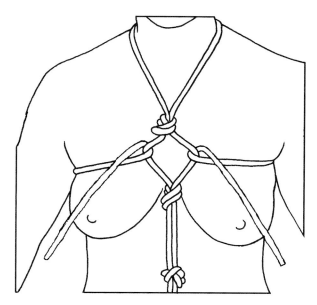

12. You'll use the free ends at the front of the body to separate the vertical lines between the pearls, thus forming the diamond shapes. Take the right free line and hook it over the right vertical line. Take the left free line and hook it over the left vertical line. Bring each of the free lines out toward the shoulders. Then drop the free lines down toward the hips and back around to the spine. This move crosses the horizontal line back over itself. This crossing creates a touch more friction in the rope, allowing the tie to hold better where it's crossed. This friction is certainly more effective with the "grabbier" organic ropes such as hemp and cotton, but adds to the overall form even with the silkier nylon lines.

13. Give a bit of a tug to make sure that the vertical lines are sufficiently separated for visual pleasure and firmness of bondage.

14. Repeat this process on the back side.

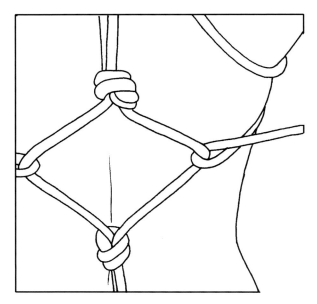

15. Return to the front side and repeat the process on the next set of vertical lines.

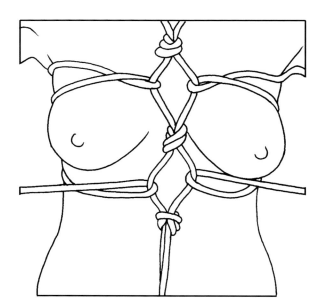

16. Continue back and front and down the body, always making sure that the ties are uniformly firm.

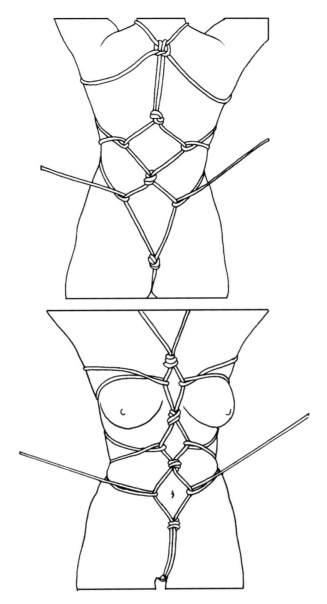

17. Tie off with simple hitches at the last dia-
    mond.

Options and Ideas: Here are some further bondage ideas to enhance the body harness!

- Tie off at the last diamond on the back and use the excess rope to bind the wrists together in the middle of the back.

- Combine it with the *Agura* (cross-legged) position. In the *Agura*, the primary tension is between the neck and the ankles, but with the Kikkou, you can distribute that tension differently. It'll make it easier on the body while being even more restrictive. Tie the body harness and then the regular *Agura*. Then run lines from the ankles to each of the pearls on the front of the torso.

- Use additional rope to tie the bottom to any chair, table, post, bed, Saint Andrew's cross or any number of other bondage furniture. Binding down the torso firmly makes the bondage very effective and increases its inescapability. It's especially key to bind down the hips. Combine this with wrist/ankle or arm/leg restraint to external bondage equipment.

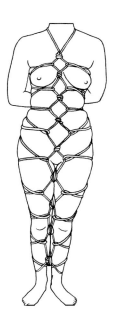

Bonus Idea: The Whole Body Tortoise Shell Harness Isn't this pretty and flattering? It'll make your bottom into a mermaid or merman! It's also extremely restrictive, as the legs are bound together. This is actually a simple variant of the knotted *Kikkou*. You'll need a lot more rope for this one.

In this harness the bottom is very vulnerable to losing balance and falling, so please make sure that he is either adequately spotted or supported. At this point you can lay him down or seat him in a chair. If you wish to keep him standing it's much safer to secure him with additional lines to weight-bearing external structures such as posts or sturdy eyebolts.

1. Instead of stopping the front side pearls at the pelvic region, continue them down the legs to the floor.

2. One of the pearls ought to be at level with the kneecaps. This will prevent the horizontal lines from pressing against the knees.

3. A loving touch is to pad between the knees and ankles. This helps to prevent chafing and more serious potential injuries.

4. At the ankle, separate the lines and bring it around on each side to the back.

5. Make another pearl at the back of the ankle and continue up the back.

6. As the legs are bound together now, make sure that the bottom is steady. Give him a secure point to hold on to if necessary.

7. Now continue with steps #9 to #17.

8. To make this position even more restrictive, I'll add rope to the loop between the legs, connecting the corresponding pearls in the front and back of the leg, binding them securely.

Step by Step: The Un-Knotted Tortoise Shell Body Harness

This is the type of tie that I used in the photo at the beginning of this chapter. While this is not entirely the traditional form, it does offer many advantages to modern sensual players. The knotted Kikkou, while traditional and attractive, relies on bulky knots that lie along the spine and breastbone. The pressure from these knots may become extremely uncomfortable over time, especially if the body is bound to any external structures. You may find yourself in the situation where you've spent time to create a beautiful bondage, only to have to untie it rapidly to rescue your bottom. For this reason, it's good to have this more contemporary variation in your repertoire. My gratitude goes out to Lou Duff for introducing me to this style!

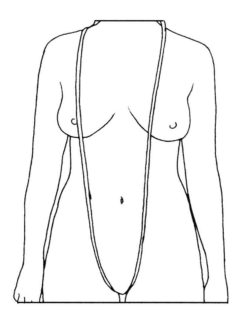

1. Fold the rope in half. Place the center point on the spine at the back of the neck with the rest of the rope over the shoulders and breasts.

3. Bring the two lines between the legs to back of the body. Whether you place a crotch knot at this point or not is up to you. See the section on crotch knots on page 27 for further discussion on this.

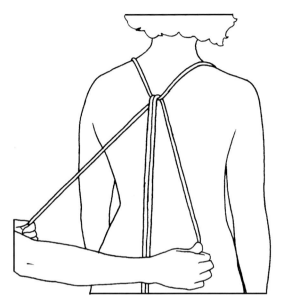

4. Take the two lines and pass the ends through the center point of the rope that rests at the back of the neck.

5. Separate the lines to the right and left sides, bringing them over the rope on the spine. Tie them with one overhand knot.

6. At this point the vertical rope base around the body should be a bit on the loose side. As the bondage continues, the horizontal lines will take up the slack considerably. If this vertical foundation is too tight, further binding might make it too uncomfortable for the bottom's pleasure or endurance. It's also difficult to create a more visually appealing series of diamonds if there's no slack in the vertical lines.

7. Separate the lines again and bring them under each arm to the front of the body.

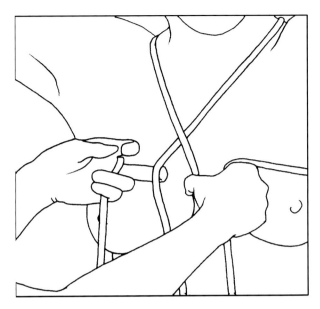

8. You'll use the free ends at the front of the body to separate the vertical lines, catching opposite lines and continuing to cross them back and forth. This is what forms the diamond shapes without the use of "pearls." Take the right free line and hook it over the *left* vertical line. Take the left free line and hook it over the *right* vertical line. Bring each of the free lines out towards the shoulders. Then drop the free lines down towards the hips and back around to the spine. This little move crosses the horizontal line back over itself. This crossing creates a touch more friction in the rope, allowing the tie to hold better where it's crossed. This friction is certainly more effective with the "grabbier" organic ropes such as hemp and cotton, but adds to the overall form even with the silkier nylon lines.

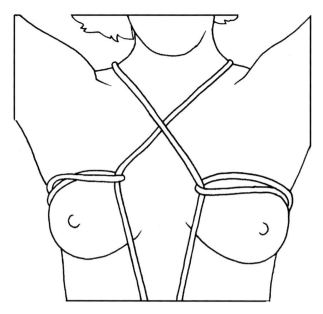

9. Give a bit of tug to make sure that the vertical lines are sufficiently separated for visual pleasure and firmness of bondage.

10. Repeat this process at on the back side.

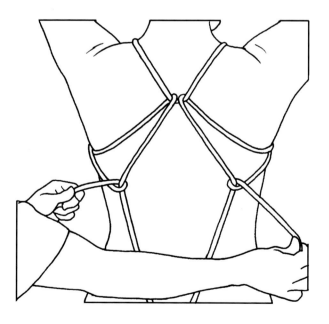

11. Return to the front side and repeat process.

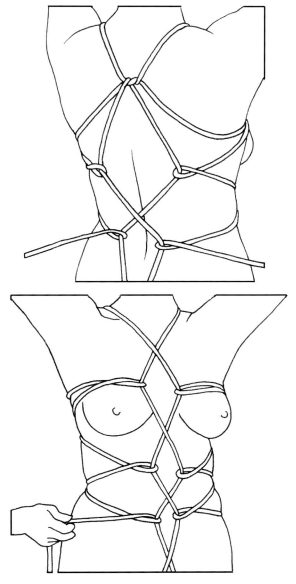

12. Continue back and front and down the body, always making sure that the ties are uniformly firm.

13. Tie off with a simple square knot after the last diamond.

14. Using this flatter, updated form of the *Kikkou* bondage, you can still enjoy the options and ideas that we discussed previously for the Knotted *Kikkou*.

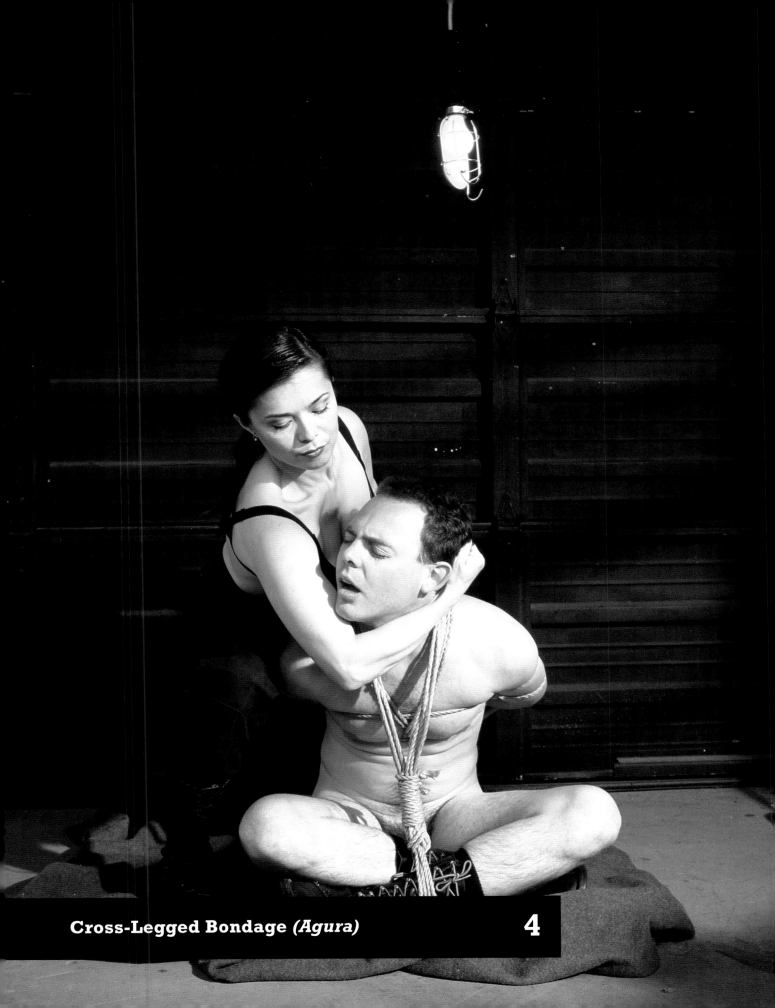

Cross-Legged Bondage *(Agura)*   **4**

Position 4. Cross-Legged Bondage (*Agura*)

I've let it be known to Sir that I'm up for a challenge tonight. As usual, he knows how to push me in just the right way. In the middle of the futon he binds me expertly into a sitting position. At first I smile defiantly back at him and wriggle to show that I'm able to endure this. He just laughs and sits back authoritatively. His confidence and my bound state made my cock throb. Eventually my smile turns to a grimace and sweat starts to build on my brow. He comes over to me and stands inches from my flushed face. I can see from the bulge in his leather pants that he's pleased with my torment and my endurance. With a casual nudge of his engineer boot he rolls me over onto my side, exposing me to all his sweetly wicked ministrations.

Fierce and challenging, the *Agura* is a traditional interrogation and detention *shibari* position.

At first sight this seems to be a relatively tolerable position – perhaps not even all that restrictive, as the bindee is not attached to any external points. This deceptive appearance may be the crucial point for fun in an erotic fantasy interrogation or captivity scene. The bottom who likes to be playfully defiant will enjoy this challenging position!

The bent-over position creates slow strain on the body while the whole configuration makes it really impossible for the bottom to escape. About the only movement available to the bottom is to roll about, which in the end only emphasizes his general helplessness and may even enhance his sense of vulnerability and exposure.

For erotic play combined with captive fantasy and masochism, this position is wonderful. Bind the bottom into captivity using the *Agura*. Then roll him to one side or another to expose his aroused and now fully accessible sex. He is at your mercy for deep pleasure or delightful torment!

When rolling him back, make certain that there's plenty of padding to alleviate the pressure on his bound wrists. I would caution against rocking him forward in a way that puts most of the pressure on the bent head and neck. This movement could be really hazardous.

As discussed in the previous position, combining this with the *Kikkou*, or Tortoise Shell, increases its effectiveness and visual appeal. Adding rope from the ankles to the pearls will help to distribute the pressure on the back of the neck and enhance the restrictiveness.

Step by Step: Cross-Legged Bondage *(Agura)*

1. Bind the wrists with the Arm and Chest *(Ushirote munenawa)* or the Tortoise Shell *(Kikkou)* combined with a wrist tie.

2. Assist the bottom down to a seated position, and make him sit with his ankles crossed.

3. Fold another rope in half. Wrap the ankles with the rope a few times forming a band, leaving the center loop hanging about 8 to 10 inches from the ankles.

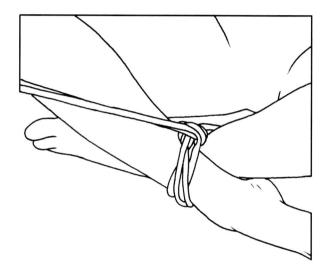

4. Wrap the line with the center loop around the ankle band, cinching the band together between the ankles. (This binding is similar to the one with which you started the Arm and Chest Bondage – see p. 72.)

5. Tie the loop and the free ends into a square knot, granny knot or series of several half hitches.

6. You should be left with an inch or two of the loop end showing and most of the free ends hanging loose. This tie is your ankle quick release. Should the feet lose circulation or get tingly, you can effortlessly untie the ankles. It also adds psychological drama to the bondage, as the bottom can see the knot that would free him in front of him, but can't quite get to it. If he is extremely flexible and you suspect he might be able to undo a simple overhand knot with his fingers or teeth, then you may want to use a series of half hitches... even the cleverest of escape artists tends to get discouraged by these after the initial challenge.

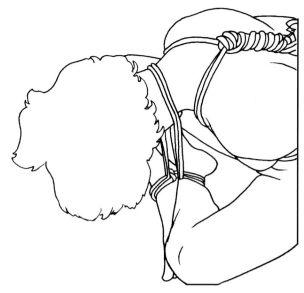

7. Take the free end of the rope and wrap it over the back of the neck, then return it to the ankle bondage. Run the free rope through the ankle bondage. Gently tug the rope to bring the body down toward the feet to an angle you desire and the bottom can hold relatively comfortably. It's a loving touch on the part of the dominant to pad the back of the neck to reduce the potential for chafing or other injury.

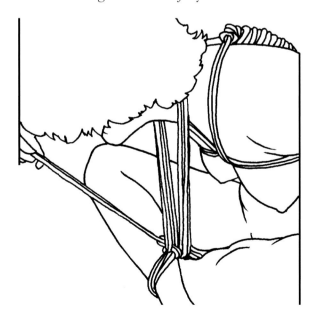

8. Repeat the process around the neck a few more times.

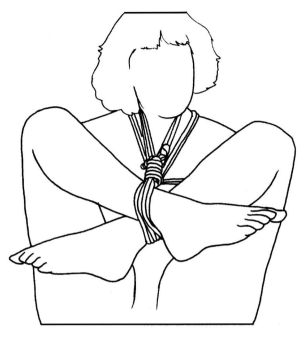

9. After the last pass through the ankle bondage, use the two free lines as one to coil around all the ropes going up to the neck.

10. When there's three or four inches remaining on the free ends, separate them. Pass one of the free ends between the neck ropes. Now you have two free lines headed in opposite directions. You can now tie a simple square knot to finish the *Agura*.

Options and Ideas:

- Instead of wrapping the rope from the ankles around the neck, wrap it around the shoulders. It'll reduce the stress on the neck and the body can move a bit more.

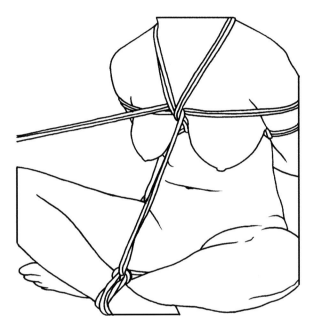

- Instead of using the neck rope, take the free lines from the ankle to the chest knot in either the Basic Breast Bondage *(Ushirote munenawa)* or the Tortoise Shell *(Kikkou)*. This is still restrictive, yet reduces the risk to the neck. With either of these first two options, the head can move relatively freely, making the face and mouth more available for sex play.

- For a heavier bondage scene combine the full form with additional lines running to the *Kikkou*, as discussed at the beginning of this chapter.

- Add the Open Leg Crab *(Kaikyaku kani)* before the ankles are bound.

- Slide a dowel or bamboo rod in the crook of the arm behind the back for even greater restriction.

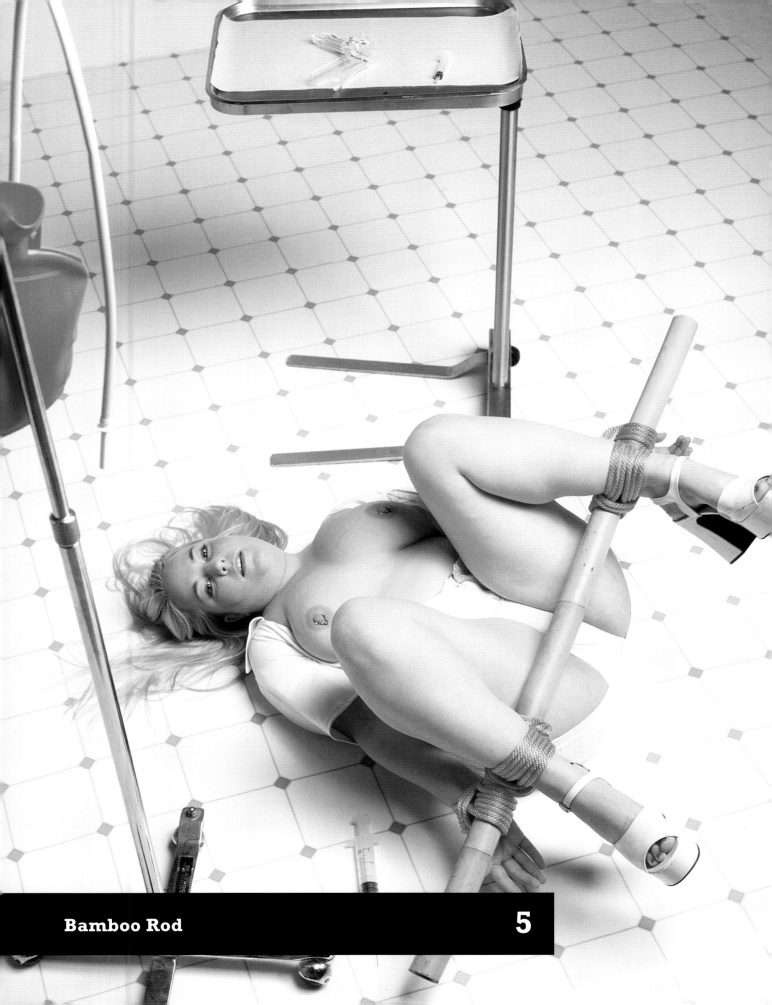

Bamboo Rod

5

Position 5. Bamboo Rod

I'm your willing pleasure-toy tonight. You've bent me this way and that. Now you've got me: I'm face down in the carpet with my legs spread before you and bound to this rod. The bamboo's coolness is a relief to my flushed skin. My breasts press into the floor with hardened nipples scraping into the carpet with each heavy breath I take. My sex is wet with desire and anticipation. My back arches to present my body to you in the most pleasing manner to you. Oh, touch me, please touch me and relieve me of this fire burning inside of me!

The use of bamboo in bondage is as culturally natural to the Japanese as using rope in bondage. It's a traditional building and crafts material that used to grow abundantly across most of the country. Aside from its simple use, as discussed here and in various parts of this book, it's also used in more elaborate bondage and even to build suspension structures. We'll save the more complicated forms for another book.

This position is the simple and elegant solution to the question of how to create an immobilizing yet sexually accessible bondage. It's also visually pleasing to the top. This makes this form one of my personal favorites!

This particular position is an example of an extremely simple yet elegant and effective form of bondage. It's also a very sexual position that allows for easy access regardless of the gender of the bottom. This position is also perfect for those whose sexual arousal is enhanced by the emotional state of vulnerability, exposure and erotic humiliation.

While technically uncomplicated, this is an extremely effective position. It's surprising how restrictive it is. Once bound in this position face-up, it's quite difficult to move to the face-down position and vice versa. I recommend that you decide in advance which position you prefer and begin the bondage in that position. If you want her on her back or face-up, start that way; if you want to have her face down, begin binding with her kneeling and then bend her down to the face-down position.

When time comes to undo her bondage, simply loosen the ropes and slide out the bamboo. The speed and ease in the untying from such an effective bondage can surprise and impress the bottom as well as being easy on the top after a fun scene.

The longer the bamboo is, the harder it will be for the bottom to move, as the excess length of the rod acts as a counter-pressure to any attempts at movement.

I have purchased my bamboo at landscaping suppliers, gardening stores and dry-goods dealers that sell silk flowers and other interior decorating raw materials. Whether you choose to use a traditional bamboo rod, wood, metal or some other dowel-like form, make sure that the surface is smooth enough to avoid splinters. Make certain too that it is strong enough not to snap while in use.

I hope that you'll also find creative new ways to incorporate the bamboo rod to enhance your *shibari!*

Step by Step: The Simple Bamboo Rod

1.   Have the bottom sit with her legs in front
     of her and her knees bent up. Place her arms
     before her with the wrists near the ankles.
     You may choose to place both wrists out-
     side or inside the legs. In general I have
     found it best to choose one or the other but
     not to mix them. For the sake of this in-
     struction, let's assume that you place her
     wrists outside the ankles.

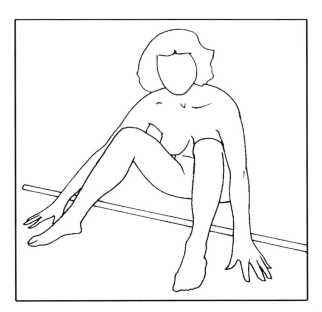

2.   Place the bamboo under the knees, just be-
     hind the ankle and under the wrist.

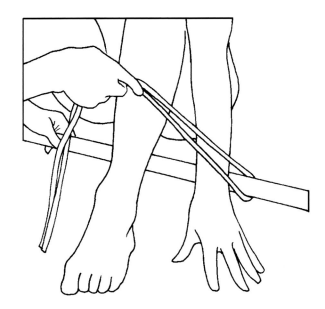

3.   Fold the first rope in half. Hook the center loop over the bamboo and slide it next to the wrist.

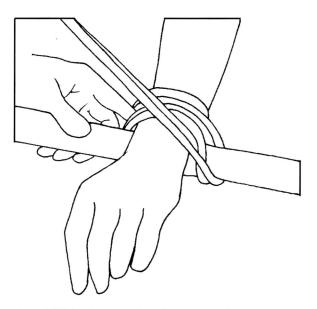

4.   With the two free lines together, pass it over the wrist and hook it over the bamboo on the other side of the wrist. Bring the rope up from under the bamboo and pass it over the wrist again.

5. Continue to wrap the wrist to the bamboo in this manner. Wrap as often as you desire, creating a band. Leave a gap between the bamboo and the wrist.

6. The last time you hook over the bamboo, instead of bringing it back over the wrist pass it under the wrist. Now wrap the rope around the band between the wrist and bamboo. This will take up the slack and secure the wrists fully to the bamboo.

8. Once you've wrapped enough to take up slack and secure the wrist, pass the free end of the rope over the ankle next to the now bound wrist. Leave a gap between the wrist and ankle so there's room to get to the bamboo.

9. The easy way to remember where to place the rod relative to the ankle is that the rod needs to rest against the Achilles tendon. The heel and calf form a natural hollow where the rod rests well without bruising the delicate top of the foot or the bony shin.

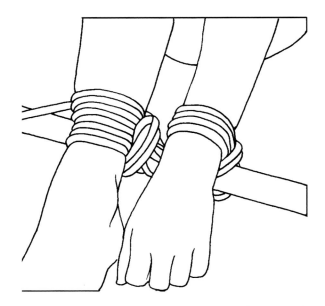

10. Pass the rope over the ankle and under the bamboo, hooking the bamboo and letting the rope come out above the rod.

11. Pass the rope over the ankle and repeat the process, forming a band joining the rod and ankle. Leave a gap between the bamboo and the ankle.

11. Secure the bamboo to the ankle as you did with the wrist. The last time you hook over the bamboo, instead of bringing it back over the ankle pass it under the ankle. Now wrap the rope around the band between the ankle and bamboo. This will take up the slack and secure the ankle fully to the bamboo.

12. Tie the rope off to the bamboo with a couple of half hitches.

13. Repeat stop 1 to 12 on the other side.

Options and Ideas:

- You can simply wrap the excess rope around the bamboo to eliminate the loose ends.

- You may also choose to secure to loose ends to an external structure.

- Or tie the loose ends from left side to the right, forming a rope triangle over the bamboo. Now you can use this rope triangle to lift up the arms and legs to a partial suspension, rolling her onto her back, exposing the sex and enhancing vulnerability. I strongly caution you against using this bamboo as the point for full suspension, as that may lead to dislocated joints.

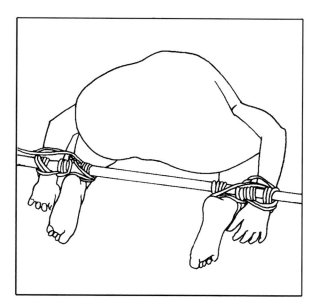

- For the face-down position, start with the bottom in a kneeling position and bind each of her ankles to the rod first, followed by each wrist. Make sure that the bamboo is placed on **top** of the ankle in this situation.

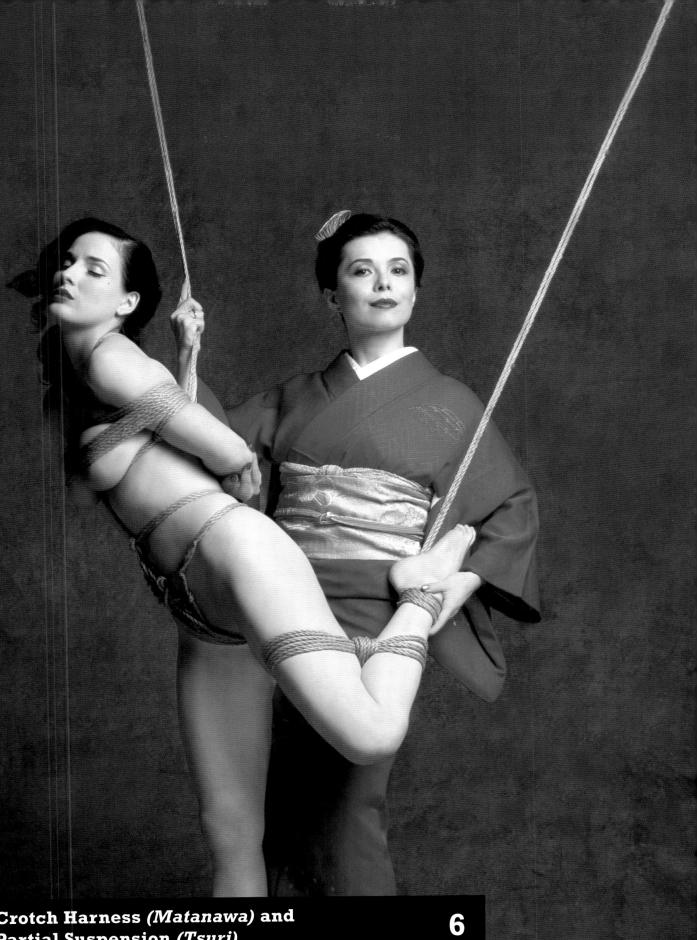

**Crotch Harness *(Matanawa)* and
Partial Suspension *(Tsuri)***

6

Position 6.
Crotch Harness *(Matanawa)* and
Partial Suspension *(Tsuri)*

With his arms bound firmly behind his back and his heart sinking deeper into submission he's ready for the next step. A quick crotch harness frames his excited cock beautifully. I've secured the heavy rope along his back to the hook in the ceiling. I tug on the rope, bringing him to his toes. He gets even harder! Carefully I tie the end off to his back with several hitches, tugging a few times to check that it's secure. I flash a big grin at him as I tie a separate band around each of his ankles. Remembering that he's right-footed, I take the rope from his right foot and start to pull it back gently. I feel the resistance. Then in one swift pull I yank it out from under him. In a rush his body tilts forward and he gasps. Then he realizes that he's still, somehow, standing. I tug on the leg leash to remind him just how vulnerable he is and just how much he is my sweet toy!

This asymmetrical position is another classic of traditional *shibari*. *Tsuri* simply means to hang, and it indicates a wide range of full and partial suspension bondage. This pose is both visually stunning and psychologically effective. The sweeping line of the body is breathtaking.

The ropes shown around the model's breasts and hips in this photo are not directly relevant to this position; I added them for decorative and sensual effect. As your Japanese bondage skills grow you'll find yourself becoming increasingly able to create your own poses, patterns and special effects as well.

I suggest you wait until you've become skilled and comfortable with the bondage techniques we've already described before you try this one. Since the bindee doesn't have the use of both feet, she is off-balance and physically vulnerable. This is not the time to have a knot fail!

You will need at least four lengths of rope for this position: one for the arm and chest harness, one to attach the arm and chest harness to the overhead attachment point for greater physical stability and safety, one for the leg tie, and one for the ankle tie. If you want to add the breast and genital wraps I've shown here, you will need extra lengths for these.

This position may be extremely physically demanding for some people. There will be more pressure placed on the upper arm bondage than in other positions, so be extra mindful of the bottom's circulation and state of well-being. Be prepared to bring her out of this position quickly if necessary. When you do this, make sure that the suspended leg is the first rope released. Once both feet are firmly on the floor, then she will feel more stable and you'll be able to make any further adjustments as necessary. As discussed before, make sure that the bottom understands her responsibility to give you good feedback in play.

Step by Step: Simple Crotch Harness *(Matanawa)*

A crotch harness may be tied alone or in conjunction with other ties. It's a great place to start genital play, a fantastic way to make both male and female bottoms achingly aware of their aroused desire and genitals. The crotch harness also serves as a great anchoring point for further bondage, such as the hogtie shown in Position 7.

Placing a crotch knot may be a fun option. Take a look at the discussion on crotch knots on page 27. Of course the crotch harness is a great way to hold a vibrator in place (page 28) or to make an impromptu dildo harness.

Here's one simple crotch harness that can be tied alone.

1.   Fold the rope in half.

2.   Place the center loop on the stomach at about waist level.

3.   Holding the center loop in place, wrap the doubled rope around the waist. This line needs to be snug but not tight.

4.   Bring the rope back around to the front.

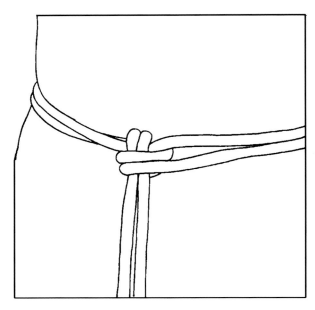

5.   Bring the rope end through the center loop and tie it off with a hitch.

6.   Run the two lines down to the crotch. Make an overhand, square or figure-eight knot. If this is on a male, place this above the base of the penis. If female, then place it above the pelvic mound.

7.   Run the ropes between the legs, making sure to keep the ropes from twisting between the legs. Also make sure that you don't catch or pinch the skin of the labia or scrotum. At this point you may want to decide about the placement of a crotch knot.

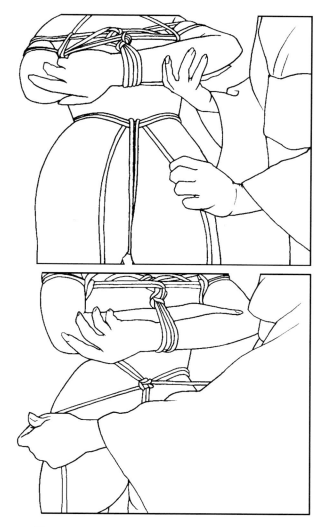

8. Bring the ropes up and over the waist rope. Then hitch it over the waist rope and tie it off in front in an overhand knot.

9. Separate the lines and let one go right and other left, and move them around to the front of the body.

10. Hook each of these ropes over and under the nearest vertical line that runs from the waist to the crotch. Tug gently to form a diamond at the lower belly. Adjust the tension of the diamond here as necessary.

11. Take the lines and run them to the right and left, taking them to the backside again.

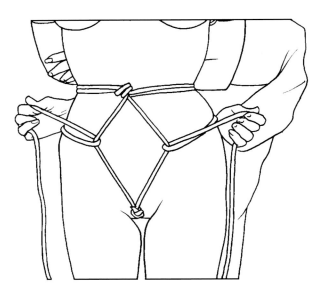

12. Hook each of these ropes over and under the nearest vertical line that runs from the back waist along the spine to the crotch. Tug gently to form a diamond at the lower back. Adjust the tension of the diamond here as necessary.

13. Tie each rope off with a hitch.

Step by Step: Partial Suspension *(Tsuri)*

We'll limit our discussion here of suspension bondage to partial suspension. Full suspension requires a level of experience that's beyond the scope of discussion for this book on basic skills.

Prepare the overhead support point in advance. This may be a horizontal beam, eyebolt, hook, suspension bar or block and tackle. Make certain that any overhead structure that you'll attach this bondage to have been tested to hold at least three times the intended bottom's body weight.

1. With the bottom seated or standing, prepare the upper body with the Arm and Chest harness *(Ushirote munenawa)* described in Position 2.

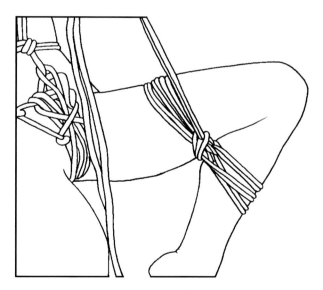

2. With the bottom seated near the overhead attachment point, prepare one leg with the Open Leg Crab *(Kaikyaku kani)* tie described in Position 1.

4. Move the submissive into position under the overhead attachment point. Since the submissive will be hopping on one foot, she will need to be carefully physically supported during this movement.

5. Slide the center loop around the knots at the middle of her back between the upper and lower horizontal bands of the Arm and Chest harness. Run the free ends through the loop.

6. Run the free ends over the overhead support that you've set up, then back down to the submissive.

7. At this point, pull the line to move the submissive's body to your desired level.

8. Tie off the free line to the same place you attached the rope, thus supporting the submissive by anchoring her to the overhead attachment. Use several hitches to make sure that the line won't untie.

9. Prepare another rope. Fold the rope in half.

10. Wrap the rope around one ankle several times forming a band, leaving 6 to 8 inches loose at the center loop.

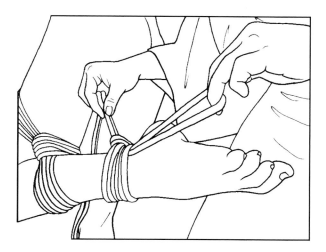

11. Run the center loop under all the ropes in the band.

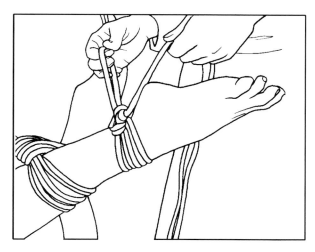

12. Use a square knot to tie off the loop end and the free end. To be extra sure, you can run the free ends through the loop, which will lock in this tie. You should be left with plenty of free rope. If not, attach more.

12. Bring up this bound leg.

12. Tie an overhand knot in the line about a foot from the ankle. We'll use this knot to tie off the rope later.

13. Attach the free rope to an overhead, weight-bearing point.

14. Bring the rope back down. Slide the free rope in the space created by the overhand knot in the line going up towards the ceiling.

15. Tie off the line with several half hitches.

Options and Ideas: This is a very physically and psychologically vulnerable position borrowed directly from medieval Japanese interrogation. It's a great situation to do male and female genital play, stimulation and torment, as the genitals are fully exposed. It's also a great position to do frontal whipping and genital flogging.

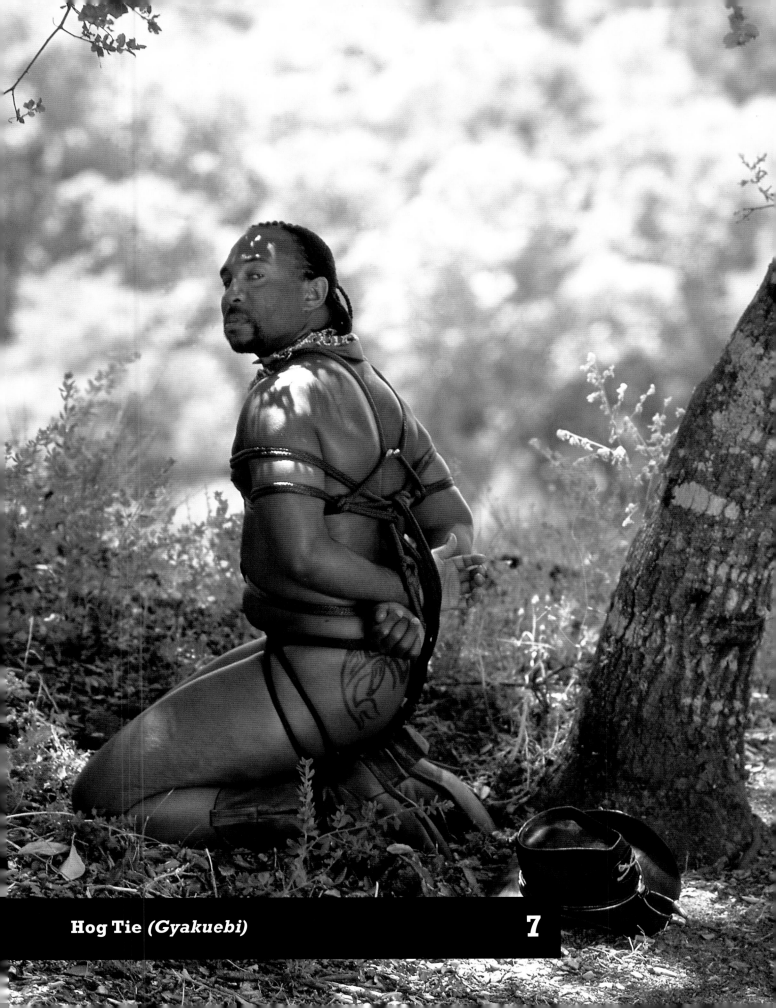

Hog Tie (Gyakuebi)   **7**

Position 7: Hog Tie *(Gyakuebi)*

Lover, let's play "cowboys" tonight! In this episode you can be the hero and I'll be the bad guy. I'll cut you off at the pass and rope you down to the ground. I'll strip you naked except your boots and hat… but I like your big gun just as it is! On your knees you go, arms corralled behind you so I can see those two pink targets waiting for my cruel attention. As I wrangle your legs back, you're my helpless captive in my mountain hideaway. I'll use you on your knees for a bit of pleasure, and then roll you onto your side to get to other parts of you. If I get a bit tired, I'll roll you over onto your belly and use you as my cowboy lounger. What would you do if I just picked you up like a trussed little calf and hauled you off to bed? Will you struggle? Will you beg? Will you be my plaything? But don't you go forgettin'… in the next episode, the hero gets to escape, capture the bad guys and save the day!

The *Gyakuebi*, or hog-tie, is another classic endurance and military interrogation position. Its dramatic look makes it a popular style for photographers and artists. It's also extremely effective in severely restricting the bottom's mobility and comfort. In fact, for many people this is a severe enough position that they can stay in it for only a limited time before it becomes excruciating and non-erotic. Therefore my advice is to not plan the entire scene around this single position, but use it as one of several positions that the bottom gets put through.

Since this position is essentially a creative combination of other basic *shibari* components, it's quite easy to shift from one position to another. For example, you can move easily to and from the hog-tie to the open-leg-crab, crossed-leg and partial suspension positions, as well as a myriad of other imaginative combinations. All of these transitions can happen without the person ever being fully out of bondage. At all times there will be a sense of sensual restriction and erotic control. Rope bondage is unique in this potential for fluidity and creativity, limited only by the players' imaginations.

The *Gyakuebi,* like so many other shibari positions such as the *Agura*, seriously restricts the mobility of the bound without external attachment points. This is an advantageous feature that will often mitigate the problems of an extremely physically difficult position. Sometimes simply moving them around or rolling them onto a different side of their body may relieve a particular strain, enabling the players to return to the pleasures of the moment. In fact, this process of moving around the hog-tied body amps ups the excitement of the scene for many players. For many bottoms it may deepen the sense of submission and sexual surrender. Conversely, many tops enjoy the visceral feeling of physical dominance. For others it's the element of struggle, roughhousing and manhandling that they find thrilling.

A comfort tip: If you're going to keep him on his knees, consider some soft and body-friendly surface for him to kneel on. Also, in this position there might be a great deal of stress on the ankles; wearing boots that cover the ankles provides a layer of protection for the bottom and a range of increased play possibilities for the top.

As an interesting aside, the Japanese name of this position means "reverse shrimp," after its arched-back body position.

Step by Step: Hog Tie *(Gyakuebi)*

1. Create the Arm and Chest Harness *(Ushi-rote munenawa)* as described in Position 2 on page 72. In the bondage shown here, I have continued the harness into a waist tie, as shown in the second Arm and Chest option on page 85.

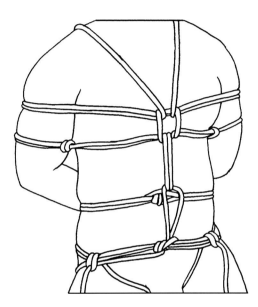

2. Create a Crotch Harness *(Matanawa)* as discussed in Position 6 on page 133. In the bondage shown here, I have passed the central point of the rope around the belly knot from the Arm and Chest Harness and then begun the Crotch Harness from the crotch knot. However, it will work equally well with the basic Crotch Harness shown in Position 6. If you've started with the standard 25 feet of rope, you will need to add another length of rope to attach to the feet in Step 6. If you want to use only one piece of rope for the lower half of the hog tie, you will need approximately 50 feet of rope.

3. Carefully bring the bottom down onto his knees. With his arms tied behind the back, his body balance is considerably off even if his legs are fully free. Holding onto the knot of ropes in the middle of his back is a good way to offer stability and support as he kneels down.

4. At this point you'll need to decide if you are going to hog-tie him while he's kneeling or lying down. This is up to you. I personally tend to like placing my bottoms on their bellies.

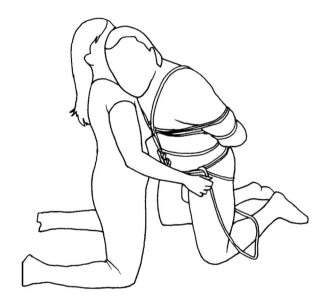

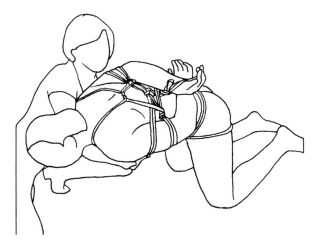

5. If you decide to lay him down read this portion. Unless you're playing on a really fluffy soft surface like a layer of comforters atop a bed, there really is no way he can safely lie down from a kneeling position on his own. You may choose to hold onto the back knot and have him lean forward, but this can also be a bit tricky unless you're very large and strong and your bottom is relatively small. As a small woman, I use my body to help guide them down to the floor. If you want to try my way, here's what you do. Sit or kneel before him and have them rest his head on your shoulder. Have him turn his head to one side or another (this keeps him from looking down at a rapidly approaching floor or from banging his nose against the floor). Then instruct him to lean into you. As he does, you slowly lower your body, essentially using your body as a buffer and guide as you lead him onto the floor. Once he is face down you can proceed with the next step.

6. If you used a short rope for the crotch harness, fold another 25-foot rope in half, and slide the halfway point into the back knot of the chest bondage, leading the free end towards the feet.

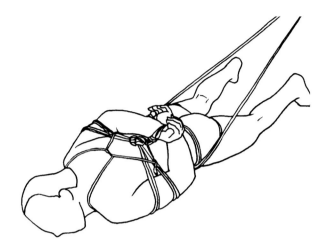

7. If you are using the ends of the crotch harness rope, as shown here, pull the ends around the hips and downward toward the feet.

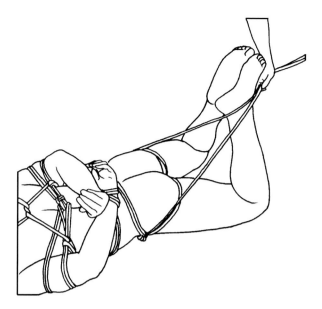

8.   Collect the feet together with one hand and bring them back up towards the thighs.

9.   With the free hand, take the two halves of the free rope as one and wrap them around the ankles. Adjust the rope as necessary to bring the legs firmly but comfortably close to the rest of the body. Wrap the ropes around the ankles until you are happy with the coverage.

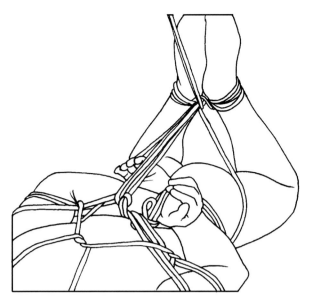

10. Run the free end over the lines that came in from the back knot. Now run the free ends between the ankles and up toward the back. You may choose to hitch it around the first line at this point.

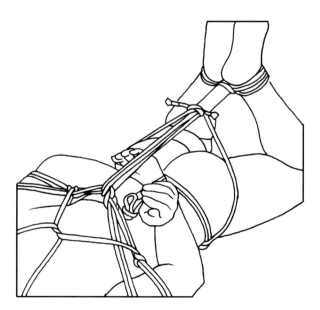

11. Return the free ends toward the back knot, wrapping them around the collected ropes to further tighten the tie.

14. You may choose to tie off here. You may also choose to tie it off along some other part of the body so Houdini-like hands can't reach the end knots.

Options and ideas: A disparity in size and strength between the top and the bottom offers some interesting possibilities...

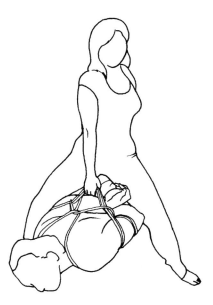

• This hog-tie turns the bottom into a very "compact" package. If the top is relatively strong, the back of the chest rope makes a convenient handle by which the bottom can be lifted and even moved.

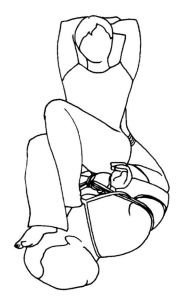

- On the other hand, if the top is smaller than the bottom, the bottom can serve as a comfy lounge chair, with his feet acting as a backrest and his head as a footrest. Stay aware of the bottom's comfort level – if he complains of being unable to breathe, it's time to stop.

Aftercare: Safe Landing After a Blissful Flight...

Some rope bondage enthusiasts compare the *shibari* experience to a journey, and often describe it as a trip or flight. Either of these is an apt analogy, as so much of bondage allows the bottom to fly free from the worries of the day and enjoy being in the moment with one's lover.

As with any journey, there's a beginning, a middle and an end. The end is just as relevant to the success of the experience as are the other components.

An entire rope scene's perceived success or failure can be colored profoundly by how well it's concluded, regardless of how wonderful the beginning and middle might have been. A jarring or poor conclusion to the scene is like crash-landing a plane after an otherwise wonderful flight. This process of successfully concluding a scene is called "Aftercare."

Since both the top and bottom are on this journey together, aftercare is just as important for the top as it is for the bottom. It may be obvious that the bottom could need safety and nurturing after a scene that may have been psychologically and physically demanding... but the same is also true for the top, who has been intensely focused and, perhaps, expressing harsh or cruel feelings (however consensual). When the top

fails to allow herself proper aftercare, she might emotionally crash from the experience even if the bottom was properly cared for.

I don't mean to worry you, but good aftercare is significant and I simply want you to be aware of its impact. To conclude a scene successfully doesn't require any special skill, but it does require common sense and compassion.

When Does a Scene End?

Sometimes a play scene will end as planned, but most often it takes unexpected and pleasurable detours. Each encounter has its natural life span, whether anticipated or not.

Sometimes the experience is so exciting that it continues on beyond what was originally planned. At other times, the players might find some particular portion of the intended activities so thrilling that the scene never goes beyond that point in the plan, and that carries the flow of the rest of the evening. Scenes may end in spicy sex or meditative quietness. Some scenes might have to be brought to conclusion more quickly than planned, due to unforeseen mood-breakers or emergencies.

The natural end to the scene usually comes when the participants are no longer able to engage in the pleasure of the shared moment. A play experience should not be pushed beyond this point. If it is, you risk turning a great scene into a less than wonderful one. The top in the scene needs to be particularly sensitive to her level of engagement in the scene and the flow of the scene as well as the bottom's pleasure feedback. It's better to leave a scene with desire peaked and all players flying high in pleasure than to force it to a place of potential boredom or resentment.

Ending a scene, much like entering the scene, is about creating a transition. It's the time necessary to come down from the remarkable journey to a comfortable equilibrium with feet planted firmly in reality. Aftercare allows for this transition. The more deep or intense the scene, the more it might have affected the participants, and the more special the aftercare might need to be.

Removing the Ropes

It's delightful if the ropes come off the skin just as mindfully as when you laid the ropes on your lover's flesh. This mindful time for removing the ropes is yet another opportunity for a new level of pleasures and sensation.

The skin wrapped in the ropes has been brought to self-awareness not commonly experienced in everyday life. The skin is fully aroused because of the ropes. At the same time, the body also habituates to the sensation of the rope embrace. Thus the rope sliding off the skin simultaneously stimulates an already aroused skin and creates the sensation of being made newly naked once again.

Experiment with how you remove the rope. Slide it off slowly or quickly, gently or roughly. Intentionally draw it across a sensitive part like nipples or genitals. Let the rope smoothly whisper along the body like a caress or brusquely tug and grab like hungry hands. After all, rope used with intent becomes an extension of the top's arms, hands, lips, tongue and desire. So use the rope as you would your hands to slowly bring the bottom down to a place of equilibrium and a sense of closure.

Sometimes I'll remove all the ropes in one continuous process. I'll keep the ropes moving in a smooth, rhythmic and constant pace, pacing the removal to slowly bring the bottom to a place of peace. At other times I'll remove one rope and let the bottom enjoy the new level of unwrappedness for a while, or I might use the interim time to play with his body and mind in other ways, before moving on to removing the next lines.

Once the Rope is Off

Once all the rope is removed, I'll generally let the bottom wallow in the state of nakedness before letting her dress. It can be such a sweet blissful twilight of pleasure for both partners, that I hate to rob my partner or myself of that time.

I find that many people are often tempted to rush from play to the next activity rather than surrender to the sweet afterglow. If there's a limited time for play, then make sure that time for proper after-care is figured into the overall plan so that it is not rushed or disregarded in the end. Use this time to savor the radiant feeling that both partners can enjoy after a good scene. There's a certain feeling of physical and emotional intoxication that comes from a delightful rope experience that's colloquially referred to as a "bondage high" or being "rope stoned." As each person experiences this state differently, they will also prefer different ways to spend the post scene time: it's wisest to ask your partner what sort of aftercare they prefer, and this goes for tops as well as bottoms. Some people like to chat after play where others prefer to spend some time in protected silence. Some might prefer to have their limbs and skin massaged where as others might find that distracting... and so on. Knowing their wind-down preferences in advance will allow you to be prepared for them.

As with many SM scenes, there's a state of physical and emotional arousal during the course of play that's accompanied by changes in body chemistry, such as a rise of endorphins or a drop in blood sugar. As the bottom emerges from the trip he might experience sudden physiological changes. He may exhibit mild shock-like symptoms, such as feeling cold, a bit dizzy or disoriented. These reactions are not uncommon and in most cases are not cause for alarm. However, you ought to deal with such physical conditions appropriately, for failing to do so may lead to more serious concerns.

The common physical aftercare techniques are really a matter of common sense.

For example, make sure that the bottom stands up or sits down slowly. Moving too quickly after a bondage scene could lead to dizziness, lightheadedness, or even fainting. You may want to give your bottom a hand in moving. Similarly, blindfolds should be removed with consideration. Don't just remove the blindfold to have the bottom open her eyes to blinding brightness. Lowering or shading the lights is one way to make the transition comfortable. You can also tell the bottom to keep her eyes shut even after the blindfold is off. This allows the eyes to accustom to the light level in the room through the eyelids.

Body temperature may change throughout the scene as well, but the change can be most noticeable at the end of the scene. Often a scene might need to be concluded quickly because someone is overheated or becomes chilled. For some the body temperature might shift only after the ropes come off. My suggestion is to deal with this as quickly as possible. If the bottom is too cold, the solution may be as simple as wrapping up the bottom warmly, snugly and lovingly, holding them and giving them a nice warm beverage. A warm bath is a nice touch as well. Be careful that the bath is not too hot, as the body's thermostat is already a bit off, so an overly hot bath could lead to lightheadedness. If he is too hot, then a cold wet towel at the back of the neck often works nicely, as can a gentle breeze over his body.

It's common to be very thirsty or hungry after a play scene. It's really considerate to have water or even electrolyte-replenishing sports drinks and snacks or energy bars ready after the scene.

The top may also be quite hungry and thirsty after a good scene, so bring enough to share!

Of course if physical problems of any variety persists long after the scene, than it's advisable to seek professional medical help. For practical advice on how to deal with SM related health issues with the medical profession, I suggest that you consult *Health Care Without Shame* by Charles Moser, Ph.D., M.D. (Greenery Press, 1999).

While bondage is a very physically sensual adventure, for many it also carries a profound emotional impact. Along with the physical comforts of aftercare, quality care for the emotional transition will make for the best landing from a great journey! Try to take the time to relax and enjoy each other's company after the scene. Don't rush off to the next scheduled activity. As mentioned earlier, some people may or may not want to talk immediately after a scene, so don't press them into conversation. It may be tempting to let enthusiasm get the better of us and to immediately ask questions on how the experience was for the other person. While some may love to share in the pleasure immediately, others prefer to save that for later. There is a time called "check-in" for talking about how the scene was. We'll discuss that in a moment.

Part of the emotional component of the aftercare is validation. Whether top or bottom, people want to know that their partner appreciated them. Tops want to know that they created an exciting scene and bottoms want to know that they bottomed well. Since both participants gave the gift of presence and vulnerability to the experience, each ought to be recognized and praised by the other. It's a gracious top who praises the bottom for his beauty in the scene. It's also the elegant bottom who thanks the top for the loving attention.

Bondage and SM scenes bring us each into the moment with sometimes emotionally and physically vulnerable play. There may be moments of insecurity that come with this kind of honesty and vulnerability. This is especially true when playing with new partners or new skills. We may have anxieties about performance, skills, desirability and other issues. The time spent in aftercare can reassure the person out of possible self-consciousness or concerns. Smiles, praise, touch, hugging, kissing and other acts of showing joy and compassion go a long way feed these emotional needs.

Ouch!

Like any physical adventure, rope bondage offers a potential for physical injuries ranging from the mild to the serious. For a discussion of basic SM and bondage-related injuries take a look at any of the good basic BDSM texts.

Here are some common concerns that come with rope bondage. I would like to thank Dr. Charles Moser for advice and updates in this arena.

1. Rope marks: These are "dents" left on the skin after the rope has been removed. These are mainly compression marks and will usually go away within an hour or two. If they're a problem for you, use padding between the rope and the skin – which is also helpful

in preventing the more significant problems discussed below.

2. Rope burns: These burns are caused by the friction of rope against skin. They are true burns – the rope creates heat as well as abrasion. They can leave scars, so your best bet is to be extra-careful to remove ropes without running them forcefully across the skin. They should be treated like any other burn: run cool water over the burned area for several minutes. Then, if the skin is broken, apply antibiotic cream a couple of times a day until the burn heals. If the skin is blistered, do not attempt to break the blister. If it seems infected or isn't healing properly, see a doctor.

3. Loss of circulation: Circulation can be cut off by overly tight ropes or by keeping limbs above the heart for too long, making it difficult for the body to pump blood into the affected part. Check the color and temperature of hands, feet and other bound parts frequently, and if they seem overly dark or cold loosen or adjust the bondage. Many bottoms cannot keep their hands over their heads for more than twenty minutes or so, while others can hold this position for much longer – err on the side of caution here. If circulation to the limb has been blocked, make sure that the limb is kept lower than the heart after the bondage comes off. Soaking it in warm (not hot) water may also help restore circulation faster. There will probably be "pins and needles" as the circulation

returns, but this isn't usually anything to worry about.

4. Nerve damage: If there is tingling or numbness in the limb afterwards – either right after the bondage comes off, or later on – that lasts for more than a few minutes, there may be damage to the nerves. This problem is particularly likely when weight or stress is placed on the wrists, so it is best to set up your bondage to avoid this situation. If you have continuing numbness, tingling, "funny feelings" or pain after bondage, see your doctor.

5. Dizziness: If the bottom feels dizzy, lightheaded or faint during or after bondage, take him down right away. Sitting with his head between his knees, or lying down with his feet up, will probably help. If a bottom loses consciousness, check his pulse and make sure he is still breathing. If breathing has stopped, if you cannot feel a pulse, if his pulse is irregular, or if he doesn't return to consciousness within five minutes or so, call 911.

The Check-In

You've had a great scene with really sweet aftercare and cool-down time. So what's left? Two more things: the check-in and making your next play date.

The check-in is that lovely conversation between the participants a day or two after play that lets each other know how they are doing and how they experienced and processed the encounter. It can be done in person or by phone, as may best suit the people involved.

The check-in is the occasion to reminisce about the pleasure shared, validate each other's contribution and gain precious information for the next encounter. It's in everyone's interest for each partner to ask the other what he or she liked about the scene and what could be improved. If something in the scene didn't work, share that as well, but do so kindly. For example, you may have found your top's harnessing skill lacking in consistent tension. Even so, telling her that "your rope sucks" is not only unkind, it's unlikely to add to her desire to play again anytime soon. Instead, perhaps phrasing the need for improvement may be the more compassionate thing to do. You may want to say something akin to "I really appreciated you tying that harness on me. I think in some spots you can tie it even tighter!" This lets the other know that

you had fun and are interested in making the experience better, while giving a clear invitation to try it again.

What if you're not interested in trying something again? Then thank them for trying it with you and then let them know that it's not an activity that you're interested in this time. Please make sure to not let the check-in sound like disapproval or blame. Also don't fail to mention some dissatisfaction in fear of hurting feelings or in hopes that the negative experience will simply go away. If it's never mentioned, there's no chance for improvement. You simply need to think of how to mention it most compassionately and constructively.

Was the experience good for you? Then now you're ready for the final step of this chapter – asking for another play date! Check-in might just be the right opportunity to ask for this or you might want to wait for another occasion. In either case, the whole journey of pleasure starts all over again as you wait in anticipation!

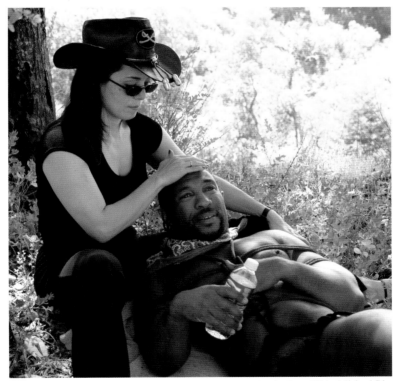

production still by Michael Blue

Tying It All Together: Conclusion

In this introductory book we've covered many of the foundations necessary to introduce you to the pleasures of Japanese rope bondage. We've discussed the history and background, eroticism, aesthetics, and scene dynamics, as well as several specific ties.

As I mentioned earlier, these positions and ties are not set in stone. There is no difinitive way in which this must be done. While Japanese rope has a long history, cultural tradition and place in the Japanese psyche, it's not a rigid and static art. It's changed and adjusted to suit the needs of the times and users, from medieval incarceration to 21st Century erotic adventures. Like the rope to the body, and like the Japanese people, it's ever adapting while maintaining a healthy respect for its foundation. Celebrate this spirit by learning the basics well and then finding your own creative expression.

As your ambassidor of kink, I hope that I've been able to open the door to new thrills and adventures for you.

Enjoy!

Fetish Diva Midori

Bibliography and Sources

The Complete Book of Knots by Geoffre Budworth ©1997 The Lyons Press

Consensual Sadomasochism: How to Talk About It and How to Do it Safely by William Henkin Ph. D. and Sybil Holiday CCSSE 1996, Daedalus Publishing Co.

Dairaku: Pleasure in the Fall photos by Takao Kawai © 1998 Japan Mix, Inc.

Jay Wiseman's Erotic Bondage Handbook by Jay Wiseman © 2000 Greenery Press

Jissan kinbaku shibarikata kyoshitsu Go Arisue ©1997 Japan Mix, Inc.

Nippon kinbaku shashinshi I, Bibliotheca Nocturna Masami Akita, Chimuo Nureki, Akio Fuji, © 1996 Jiyukokuminsha

Trans Body Bondage: Haruki Yukimura Bondage Chronicle photo by Junko Takahashi, © 1998 Wailea Publishing Co.

Yokubosuru haiheelu Doumu Kitahara © 1994 Sanichi sho

http://www.tokyo.to The Tokyo Journal, Japanese S/M parts I (10/98) and III (2/99)

http://www.webcom.com/jikatabi/hojo.html Richard Cleaver text and translations

http://www.jail-ory.com/oda/kinbaku/kinbaku.html by Hisa Oda

About the Author

Educator and writer on SM, fetish and human sexuality, Fetish Diva Midori has traveled the world presenting to universities, the SM community, media, and the greater society. Born in Japan and raised in a feminist intellectual Tokyo household, she enlisted and was subsequently commissioned as a US Army Reserves Intelligence officer while earning her psychology degree from University of California, Berkeley.

Active exploration and participation in the SM/Leather/Fetish communities, combined with numerous years as a sex educator with San Francisco Sex Information, complete the dynamic blend of experiences that give her such breadth and depth of knowledge in human erotic expression.

Midori has presented at universities, conferences, club meetings and erotic boutiques internationally. Her writings and contributions have appeared in many books and magazines, including *Wired, Esquire (UK), Skin Two* and *Playboy*. She's also appeared in many television, radio and live net programs on HBO, Playboy TV, BBC, German TV, and more. She is currently working on several books and seminar tours. She was christened "Fetish Diva" by the father of the modern primitives, Fakir Musafar.

More information about Midori, her classes and writings can be found at *http://www.fhp-inc.com*. Her website *http://www.BoundBeauty.com* offers free discussion groups for bondage tops and bottoms as well as extensive photographs of more advanced and challenging Japanese bondage styles and techniques.

About the Photographer

Craig Morey was born in 1952 in Ft. Wayne, Indiana, in the Midwestern U.S. He attended Indiana University and stued with the noted Bauhaus artist, Henry Holmes Smith. Morey's personal work with abstract and whimsical black & white nudes has garnered numerous awards, including a Special Jury Prize at the International Triennial of Photography in Friebourg, Switzerland, and First Prize at the California State Exposition. He was named one of five worldwide "Discoveries" by *Time-Life's Photography* Year 1981.

Beginning in 1988, working on assignment for *Penthouse*, Morey began creating a series of striking black & white nudes which appeared in publications in the U.S., Canada, and Europe. A hardcover monograph of selections from this *Penthouse* project, *Studio Nudes*, was published in Fall 1992. A second book of images, *Body/Expression/Silence*, was released in Japan in 1994, and another Japanese monograph, *Linea*, was published by Korinsha Press of Kyoto in 1996. Morey's newest collection, *Twentieth Century Studio Nudes*, was released in German, French and English by Glaspalast Edition of Germany in 2001.

More of Morey's work can be viewed on his website at *http://www.moreystudio.com*.

Other Books from Greenery Press

BDSM/KINK

The Bullwhip Book
Andrew Conway — $11.95

The Compleat Spanker
Lady Green — $12.95

Family Jewels: A Guide to Male Genital Play and Torment
Hardy Haberman — $12.95

Flogging
Joseph W. Bean — $11.95

Jay Wiseman's Erotic Bondage Handbook
Jay Wiseman — $16.95

KinkyCrafts: 99 Do-It-Yourself S/M Toys
Lady Green — $16.95

The Loving Dominant
John Warren — $16.95

Miss Abernathy's Concise Slave Training Manual
Christina Abernathy — $12.95

The Mistress Manual: The Good Girl's Guide to Female Dominance
Mistress Lorelei — $16.95

The Sexually Dominant Woman: A Workbook for Nervous Beginners
Lady Green — $11.95

SM 101: A Realistic Introduction
Jay Wiseman — $24.95

GENERAL SEXUALITY

Big Big Love: A Sourcebook on Sex for People of Size and Those Who Love Them
Hanne Blank — $15.95

The Bride Wore Black Leather... And He Looked Fabulous!: An Etiquette Guide for the Rest of Us
Andrew Campbell — $11.95

The Ethical Slut: A Guide to Infinite Sexual Possibilities
Dossie Easton & Catherine A. Liszt — $16.95

A Hand in the Bush: The Fine Art of Vaginal Fisting
Deborah Addington — $13.95

Health Care Without Shame: A Handbook for the Sexually Diverse and Their Caregivers
Charles Moser, Ph.D., M.D. — $11.95

Look Into My Eyes: How to Use Hypnosis to Bring Out the Best in Your Sex Life
Peter Masters — $16.95

Phone Sex: Oral Thrills and Aural Skills
Miranda Austin — $15.95

Sex Disasters... And How to Survive Them
C. Moser, Ph.D., M.D. and J. Hardy — $16.95

Turning Pro: A Guide to Sex Work for the Ambitious and the Intrigued
Magdalene Meretrix — $16.95

When Someone You Love Is Kinky
Dossie Easton & Catherine A. Liszt — $15.95

FICTION

The 43rd Mistress: A Sensual Odyssey
Grant Antrews — $11.95

... But I Know What You Want: 25 Sex Tales for the Different
James Williams — $13.95

Haughty Spirit
Sharon Green — $11.95

Love, Sal: letters from a boy in The City
Sal Iacopelli, ill. Phil Foglio — $13.95

Murder At Roissy
John Warren — $15.95

The Warrior Within
Sharon Green — $11.95

The Warrior Enchained
Sharon Green — $11.95

Please include $3 for first book and $1 for each additional book with your order to cover shipping and handling costs, plus $10 for overseas orders. VISA/MC accepted. Order from:

greenery press
3403 Piedmont Ave. #301, Oakland, CA 94611
toll-free 888/944-4434   http://www.greenerypress.com